OSCE in Neonatology
A Guide Book

OSCE in Neonatology
A Guide Book

Editors-in-Chief

Srinivas Murki
MD DNB DM(Neo)
Senior Consultant
Fernandez Hospital
Hyderabad, Telangana, India

Rhishikesh Thakre
MD DNB DM(Neo) DCH FCPS FIAP
Consultant Neonatologist
Director
Neo Clinic and Hospital
Aurangabad, Maharashtra, India

Foreword
Praveen Kumar

An Official Publication of Indian Academy of Pediatrics
NEONATOLOGY CHAPTER

The Health Sciences Publisher
New Delhi | London | Panama

Jaypee Brothers Medical Publishers (P) Ltd

Headquarters

Jaypee Brothers Medical Publishers (P) Ltd
4838/24, Ansari Road, Daryaganj
New Delhi 110 002, India
Phone: +91-11-43574357
Fax: +91-11-43574314
Email: jaypee@jaypeebrothers.com

Overseas Offices

J.P. Medical Ltd
83 Victoria Street, London
SW1H 0HW (UK)
Phone: +44 20 3170 8910
Fax: +44 (0)20 3008 6180
Email: info@jpmedpub.com

Jaypee-Highlights Medical Publishers Inc
City of Knowledge, Bld. 235, 2nd Floor, Clayton
Panama City, Panama
Phone: +1 507-301-0496
Fax: +1 507-301-0499
Email: cservice@jphmedical.com

Jaypee Brothers Medical Publishers (P) Ltd
17/1-B Babar Road, Block-B, Shaymali
Mohammadpur, Dhaka-1207
Bangladesh
Mobile: +08801912003485
Email: jaypeedhaka@gmail.com

Jaypee Brothers Medical Publishers (P) Ltd
Bhotahity, Kathmandu
Nepal
Phone: +977-9741283608
Email: kathmandu@jaypeebrothers.com

Website: www.jaypeebrothers.com
Website: www.jaypeedigital.com

Inquiries for bulk sales may be solicited at: jaypee@jaypeebrothers.com

OSCE in Neonatology: A Guide Book

First Edition: **2018**

ISBN 978-93-5270-105-6

Printed at Sanat Printers

Editorial Board

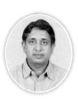
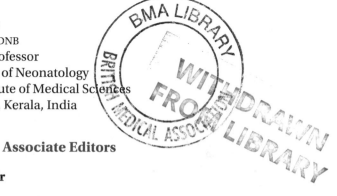
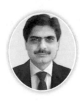
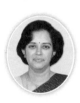

Editorial Advisory Board

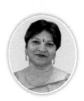

Office Bearers

Neonatology Chapter of Academy of Pediatrics

Office Bearers 2017–18

Chairperson	:	Dr Sanjay Wazir
Hon. Secretary	:	Dr Naveen Bajaj
Treasurer	:	Dr Nandkishor Kabra
Joint Secretary	:	Dr Rajesh Kumar
Imm. Past Chairperson	:	Dr Rhishikesh Thakre

Executive Members

East Zone	:	Dr Arjit Mohapatra, Dr Vinod Kumar
West Zone	:	Dr Ashish Mehta, Dr Sanjay Ghorpade
North Zone	:	Dr Deepak Chawla, Dr Kamal Arora
Central Zone	:	Dr Basawaraj T, Dr Ravi Shankar K
South Zone	:	Dr Suman Rao, Dr VC Manoj

Indian Academy of Pediatrics

Office Bearers 2017

President	:	Dr Anupam Sachdeva
President Elect, 2017	:	Dr Santosh T Soans
Vice President	:	Dr Mahaveer Prasad Jain
Imm. Past President	:	Dr Pramod Jog
Secretary General	:	Dr Bakul J Parekh
Treasurer	:	D Sandeep Bapu Kadam
Editor-in-Chief, IP	:	Dr Dheeraj Shah
Editor-in-Chief, IJPP	:	Dr NC Gowrishankar
Joint Secretary	:	Dr Ajay Gambhir

Contributors

Adhisivam B DCH DNB
Associate Professor
Department of Neonatology
Jawaharlal Institute of Postgraduate
Medical Education and Research
Puducherry, India
E-mail: adhisivam1975@yahoo.
co.uk

AK Rawat MD
Professor and Head
Department of Pediatrics
Bundelkhand Medical College
Sagar, Madhya Pradesh, India
E-mail: drakrawat01@rediffmail.
com

Amrit Jeevan DCH MD
Surya Mother and Child Super
Speciality Hospital
Mumbai, Maharashtra, India
E-mail: dramritjeevan@gmail.com

Anil Kumar MD
Consultant Neonatologist
Cloud Nine Hospital
Gurugram, Haryana, India
E-mail: dranil_kr@rediffmail.com

Anjali Kulkarni MD
Former Head
Department of Pediatrics and
Neonatology
Sir HN Reliance Foundation
Hospital
Mumbai, Maharashtra, India
E-mail: dr.kulkarnianjali@gmail.
com

Anu Sachdeva MD DNB (Pediatrics)
MNAMS DM (Neonatology)
Assistant Professor
Department of Pediatrics
All India Institute of Medical
Sciences
New Delhi, India
E-mail: dranuthukral@gmail.com

Anuradha Murki MS
Assistant Professor
Department of Obstetrics and
Gynecology
Kamineni Academic Institute and
Research Center
Hyderabad, Telangana, India
E-mail: dogiparthi_anu@yahoo.com

Archana Kadam MD DNB
Developmental Pediatrician
KEM Hospital and Jehangir Hospital
Pune, Maharashtra, India
E-mail: dr.archana.ped@gmail.com

Ashish Jain DM (Neo) MD
Assistant Professor
Department of Neonatology
Maulana Azad Medical College
New Delhi, India
E-mail: neoashish2008@gmail.com

Asim Kumar Mallick MD
Professor and In-Charge, Neonatal
Unit
Department of Pediatrics
NRS Medical College and Hospital
Kolkata, West Bengal, India
E-mail: asim_mallick2004@yahoo.
com

Atul Kulkarni MD
Assistant Professor
Ashwini Rural Medical College and
Hospital
Solapur, Maharashtra, India
E-mail: dratulkulkarni@rediffmail.
com

Bhavani Kalavalapalli MRCPCH
CCT FRCPCH
Consultant Pediatrician and
Neonatologist
Director
Institute of Diabetes, Endocrinology
and Adiposity Centres

Hyderabad, Telangana, India
E-mail: bhavani_kalavalapalli@
yahoo.co.uk

Brajesh Jha DM
Senior Resident (Neo)
Department of Neonatology
Maulana Azad Medical College
New Delhi, India
E-mail: docbkjha@gmail.com

Chandrasekharam
MCH(Paediatric Surgery)
Pediatric Surgeon
Ankura Hospital
Hyderabad, Telangana, India
E-mail: vvsssekharam@yahoo.co.in

Deepak Niraj DM (Neo) MD
Senior Consultant
BJ Wadia Children Hospital
Mumbai, Maharashtra, India
E-mail: drndipak@gmail.com

Deepak Sharma DNB (Neo) MD
Consultant Neonatologist
Neo Clinic
Jaipur, Rajasthan, India
E-mail: dr.deepak.rohtak@gmail.
com

Dhanya Dharmapalan MD
Consultant Pediatrician
Apollo Hospital
Navi Mumbai, Maharashtra, India
E-mail: drdhanyaroshan@gmail.
com

Dinesh Chirla MD DM MRCPCH
Director
Rainbow Children Hospital
Hyderabad, Telangana, India
E-mail: dchirla@gmail.com

Femitha P DM (Neo) MD
Associate Consultant
Department of Neonatology
Kerala Institute of Medical Sciences
Thiruvananthapuram, Kerala, India
E-mail: femi_shifas@yahoo.com

**Haribalakrishna
Balasubramanian** DM (Neo) MD
Surya Children Hospital
Mumbai, Maharashtra, India
E-mail: doctorhbk@gmail.com

Hemasree Kandraju MD DNB(Neo)
Consultant Neonatologist
Fernandez Hospital
Hyderabad, Telangana, India
E-mail: drhema4@gmail.com

J Kumutha MD DCH
Professor and Head
Department of Neonatology
Saveetha Medical College
Chennai
Tamil Nadu, India
E-mail: dr_kumutha@yahoo.com

Kanishka Das MS MCH
Professor
Department of Pediatric Surgery
St John's Hospital
Bengaluru, Karnataka, India
E-mail: kanishkadas@hotmail.com

Kanithi Ravishankar DM (Neo) MD
Director
Sowmya Children's Hospital
Hyderabad, Telangana, India
E-mail: ravineonatologist@gmail.
com

LS Deshmukh DM (Neo) MD
Professor and Head
Department of Neonatology
Government Medical College and
Hospital
Aurangabad, Maharashtra, India
E-mail: deshmukhls@yahoo.com

Madhavi Shelke MD
Fellowship in Pediatric Neurology
Consultant Pediatric Neurologist
ICON Centre for
Child Neurodevelopment
Aurangabad, Maharashtra, India
E-mail: madhavishelke@yahoo.com

Madhavi V MD
Clinical Geniticist
Fernandez Hospital
Hyderabad, Telangana, India
E-mail: damamadhavai@gmail.com

Mangala Bharathi S MD DM(Neo) DNB
Associate Professor
Department of Neonatology
Institute of Child Health and
Hospital for Children
Madras Medical College
Chennai, Tamil Nadu, India
E-mail: drmangalabharathi@gmail.
com

**Manigandan
Chandrasekaran** MD
Department of Neonatology
Saveetha Medical College
Chennai, Tamil Nadu, India

Mehul Shah MD (Ped) DCH (Bom) MD
(USA) DABPN (USA)
Consultant Pediatric Nephrologist
Apollo Health City and Little Stars
Childrens Hospital
Hyderabad, Telangana, India
E-mail: mehulashah@hotmail.com

Mohit Sahni MBBS DCH DNB(Ped)
Fellowship Neonatology and
Neonatal Cardiology
Sydney (Australia) and
Toronto (Canada)
Director NICU and Accedemics
Consultant Neonatologist and
Neonatal Cardiologist
Nirmal Hospital Pvt Ltd.
Surat, Gujarat, India
E-mail: mohitsahni2505@gmail.com

Monika Kaushal DM (Neo) MD
Visiting Fellowship RCPCH
Head
Department of Pediatrics and
Neonatology
Zulekha Hospital
Dubai, UAE
E-mail: mkaushal@zulekhahospitals.
com

Murlidhar D Mahajan MD DCH
DNB MNAMS
Consulting Metabolic Specialist
Jupiter Hospital
Mumbai, Maharashtra, India
E-mail: drmurlidhar@rediffmail.com

N Chandra Kumar MD DNB
MNAMS DM (Neonatology) DNB (Neo)
Director
Cloud Nine
Chennai, Tamil nadu, India
E-mail: drchandrakumar@gmail.
com

Nageshwar Rao DM MD
Chief
Division of Pediatric Cardiology
Care Hospital
Hyderabad, Telangana, India
E-mail: drkoneti@yahoo.com

Nandkishor S Kabra DM (Neo)
MD (Ped) DNB (Ped) MSc (Clinical
Epidemiology)
Director, Neonatal Intensive Care
Unit
Surya Children's Medicare Pvt Ltd
Mumbai, Maharashtra, India
E-mail: nskabra@gmail.com

Naveen Bajaj DM (Neo) MD
Consultant Neonatologist
Department of Neonatology
Deep Hospital
Ludhiana, Punjab, India
E-mail: bajajneo@gmail.com

Naveen Jain DM (Neo) MD DNB
Associate Professor
Department of Neonatology
Kerala Institute of Medical Sciences
Thuruvananthapuram, Kerala, India
E-mail: naveen_19572@hotmail.com

Nitasha Bagga MD
Consultant
Rainbow Children Hospital
Hyderabad, Telangana, India
E-mail: nitashabagga@gmail.com

Pankaj Bhansali MD
Consultant Nephrologist
Niramay Children Hospital
Aurangabad, Maharashtra, India
E-mail: drpbhansali@gmail.com

Pradeep Suryawanshi MD DCH
(Sydney)
Fellowship in Neontal Perinatal
Medicine (Australia)
Professor and Head
Department of Neonatology
BVU Medical College
Pune, Maharashtra, India
E-mail: drpradeepsuryawanshi@
gmail.com

Pradnya Deshmukh MS (Ophth)
Associate Professor
Department of Ophthalmology
MGM College and Hospital
Aurangabad, Maharashtra, India
E-mail: pradnya_kerkar@yahoo.co.in

Prashant P Patil MD (Peds) PDCC ESPE
Consultant Pediatric and Adolescent
Endocrinologist and Diabetologist
Rainbow Pediatric Multispeciality
Clinic
Mumbai, Maharashtra, India
E-mail: dr_prash4u@yahoo.com

Prashantha YN MD DM
Senior Resident
Department of Neonatology
St John's Medical College Hospital
Bengaluru, Karnataka, India

Preetha Joshi MD
Fellowship in NICU, University of
Sydney and Hamilton
Fellowship in PICU, Critical Care
Transport
Cardiac ICU, University of Sydney
and Toronto
Pediatric and Neonatal Intensivist
Kokilaben Dhirubhai Ambani
Hospital
Mumbai, Maharashtra, India
E-mail: preetha.joshi@relianceada.
com

Premal Naik MS DNB (Ortho)
Department of Orthopedics
Smt SCL Hospital
Smt NHL Municipal Medical College
Ahmedabad, Gujarat, India
E-mail: premalnaik@gmail.com

Rahul Bhamkar MD
Associate Consultant
Sir HN Reliance Foundation
Hospital
Mumbai, Maharashtra, India
E-mail: Rahul.Bhamkar@rfhospital.org

Rajesh Kumar DM (Neo) MD
Director and Chief Neonatologist
Rani Hospital
Ranchi, Jharkhand, India
*E-mail: drrajeshranihospital@gmail.
com*

Rajiv Sharan DNB MNAMS
Consultant Pediatrician
Tata Motors Hospital
Jamshedpur, Jharkhand, India
E-mail: drrajeev_sharan@yahoo.com

Raktima Chakrabarti MD
Fellowship in Neonatology (Germany)
Consultant Pediatrician and
Neonatologist
Escape, Nirvana Country
Gurugram, Haryana, India
E-mail: dr_raktima@yahoo.com

Ramani Ranjan DCH MD
Fellowship in Neonatalogy
Specialist in Pediatrics and
Neonatology
Tata Main Hospital
Jamshedpur, Jharkhand, India
E-mail: dr.rranjan@tatasteel.com

Rhishikesh Thakre MD DNB
DM(Neo) DCH FCPS FIAP
Consultant Neonatologist
Director
Neo Clinic and Hospital
Aurangabad, Maharashtra, India
E-mail: rptdoc@gmail.com

Roopa Bellad MD DCH
Professor
Department of Pediatrics
Jawaharlal Nehru Medical College
Belgaum, Karnataka, India
E-mail: roopabellad@hotmail.com

Sandeep Kadam MD DM (Neo)
Senior Neonatal Consultant
KEM Hospital and Ratna Hospital
Pune, Maharashtra, India
E-mail: drsandeepkadam@gmail.com

Sandeep Patil MD DM(Neo)
Consultant Neonatologist
"Care" Advanced Neonatal Center
Nanded, Maharashtra, India
E-mail: drsandeepsudpatil@gmail.
com

Sanjay Wazir DM (Neo) MD
Director
Department of Neonatology
Cloudnine Hospital
Gurugram, Haryana, India
E-mail: swazir21@gmail.com

Smruti Patel MD
Fellowship in Pediatric Cardiology
Pediatric Cardiologist
Fortis Hospital, Deep Hospital
Ludhiana, Punjab, India
E-mail: smrutivp@rediffmail.com

Snehal Kulkarni MD DNB (Card) FACC
Chief
Division of Pediatric Cardiology
Kokilaben Dhirubhai Ambani
Hospital
Mumbai, Maharashtra, India
E-mail: kulkarnisnehal15@yahoo.
com

Snehal Thakre MS (Ophthal) DNB
Professor
Department of Ophthalmology
MGM Medical College and Hospital
Aurangabad, Maharashtra, India
E-mail: tsnehal73@gmail.com

Srinivas Murki MD DNB DM(Neo)
Senior Consultant
Fernandez Hospital
Hyderabad, Telangana, India
E-mail: srinivas_murki2001@yahoo.
com

Suman Rao PN DM (Neo) MD
Professor and Head
Department of Neonatology
St John's Medical College Hospital
Bengaluru, Karnataka, India
E-mail: raosumanv@rediffmail.com

**Surg Cmde Sheila S Mathai,
VSM** DM (Neo) MD DNB
Professor and Head
Department of Pediatrics
Armed Forces Medical College
Pune, Maharashtra, India
E-mail: sheilamathai@yahoo.com

Tanushri Mukherjee DCH DNB
IAP Neonatology Fellowship
Clinical Associate
Department of Neonatology
Kokilaben Dhirubhai Ambani Hospital
Mumbai, Maharashtra, India
E-mail: gettanushri@gmail.com

Tejopratap Oleti DM (Neo) MD
Consultant Neonatologist
Fernandez Hospital
Hyderabad, Telangana, India
E-mail: tejopratap@gmail.com

Umesh Vaidya MD
Head
Department of Neonatology
KEM Hospital
Pune, Maharashtra, India
E-mail: kemnicu@gmail.com

Vaman V Khadilkar MD DNB MRCP
(UK) DCH (London)
Consultant Pediatrician, Adolescent
Endocrinologist and Diabetologist
Jehangir Hospital, Pune
Bombay Hospital, Mumbai
Head
Division of Pediatric Endocrinology

xiv

Bharati Vidyapeeth Medical College
Pune, Maharashtra, India
E-mail: vamankhadilkar@gmail.com

VC Manoj MD
Associate Professor and Head
Department of Neonatology
Jubilee Mission Medical College
Thrissur, Kerala, India
E-mail: jubileenicu@gmail.com

Vijay Yewale MD
Consultant Pediatrician
Apollo Hospital
Navi Mumbai, Maharashtra, India
E-mail: vnyewale@gmail.com

Vikram Hirekerur MD DCH DNB
Associate Professor
Ashwini Rural Medical College and
Hospital
Solapur, Maharashtra, India
E-mail: vikram.hirekerur@yahoo.com

Vinay Joshi DM (Neo) MD
Fellowship in PICU and PCICU,
University of Toronto, Canada
Fellowship in Neonatal and
Perinatal Medicine, University of
New South Wales, Sydney, Australia
Pediatric Intensivist and
Neonatologist
Kokilaben Dhirubahai Ambani
Hospital
Mumbai, Maharashtra, India
E-mail: Vinay.Hk.Joshi@relianceada.com

Yogesh Waikar MD DNB MNAMS
PGCC
Fellow in Pediatric Gastroenterology
and Liver Transplant
Consultant Pediatric
Gastroenterologist and Hepatologist
Pedgihep Clinics
Nagpur, Mahrashtra, India
E-mail: pedgihep@yahoo.com

Foreword

Neonatal intensive care has always been a highly technology-dependent specialty. With exponential advancements in medical equipment and laboratory in recent years, the clinical skills of eliciting history, doing a systematic but meaningful examination and synthesizing the data to reach at a pathophysiological diagnosis have further dwindled. The goal behind publication of this book is to facilitate a structured and systematic approach to clinical evaluation, examination and skills essential for 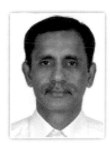 care of the sick newborn. In addition, the book also offers very useful and practical information about imaging, medications and vital statistics related to India's newborn. Divided into theme-based sections, several topics of practical and clinical relevance have been covered with focus on essential clinical skills.

Over the last decade, the Neonatology Chapter of Indian Academy of Pediatrics has taken great strides and done phenomenal work towards training and education of postgraduates, fellows and nurses in the field of neonatology. The dynamic, committed and highly motivated leadership of this chapter has mastered the art of organizing high quality workshops and conferences with pure academic focus in a short span of time. They have excelled in producing and publishing a number of hugely popular resources for everyone working for the care of newborns. *OSCE in Neonatology: A Guide Book* is another unique effort to help the postgraduates and fellows in honing their skills in neonatal medicine. OSCEs are an essential and very effective method of teaching, learning and evaluating neonatology. The book should serve as a useful resource for examiners.

I am confident this book will become an essential resource for all students, house officers, postgraduates, fellows and clinicians working in SNCUs and NICUs. The contributions of more than 60 trained neonatologists, should be able to guide readers towards optimal and rational utilization of available resources translating into better and cost-effective clinical care.

My best wishes for the success of *OSCE in Neonatology: A Guide Book*.

Praveen Kumar
Professor, Neonatal Unit
Department of Pediatrics
Post Graduate Institute of Medical Education and Research
Chandigarh, India

Preface

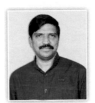

Srinivas Murki
MD DNB DM(Neo)

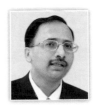

Rhishikesh Thakre
MD DNB DM(Neo) DCH FCPS FIAP

We take great pleasure and pride in offering the *OSCE in Neonatology: A guide book*. Clinical medicine is the core of patient care. History, physical examination, ordering tests and their interpretation form the foundation of this clinical medicine. Knowing the family and establishing rapport with the parents would also add value to the clinical care. In the present technology-driven neonatal care, there is tendency to ignore the core concepts and order of tests and investigations even before a detailed evaluation of the newborn. In this book, we have provided a structured approach to the newborn care with special emphasis on history, examination, interpretation of laboratory tests and tried to bridge the gap between bench and bedside.

The book has chapters on focused history, focused examination, emergency room assessment and stabilization, case scenarios, drugs, equipment, interpreting tests/results and counseling, which provide insights into clinical approach. We sincerely hope the book adds to the armamentarium of postgraduates, fellows, and students of neonatology to sharpen the skills and provide a rational clinical approach.

We are grateful to all our authors for their valuable contributions without which this book would not have seen the light of the day. We would appreciate and look forward to your feedback and comments.

We thank the office bearers of IAP Neonatology Chapter for having the faith in us. We appreciate all the support of Shri Jitendar P Vij (Group Chairman), Mr Ankit Vij (Group President), Ms Ritu Sharma (Director–Content Strategy), Ms Sunita Katla (PA to Group Chairman and Publishing Manager), Mr Manish Pahuja (General Manager–Production) for all their support to work in this project and make it a success. Without their cooperation, we could not have completed this project.

Contents

Chapter 1. Focused History Taking 1

    Instructions to Facilitator 1

    Preterm Admission at Birth 1

    Feeding History Taking 2

    Inadequate Breast Milk 4

    Respiratory Distress 4

    Shock 5

    Hypoglycemia 5

    Jaundice 6

Chapter 2. Focused Clinical Examination 8

    Well Baby Examination 8

    Breastfeeding 10

    Weight, Length and Occipitofrontal Circumference (OFC)

    Measurement 11

    Capillary Refill Time 13

    Blood Pressure Measurement by Oscillometry 14

    Developmental Dysplasia of Hip 14

    Jaundice 16

    Moro Examination 17

    Popliteal Angle.. 18

    Heel to Ear Examination 19

    Scarf Sign 19

    Assessment of Shoulder Tone 20

    Palmar Grasp Reflex 22

    Plantar Grasp Reflex 23

    Asymmetric Tonic Neck Reflex 24

    Denver Developmental Screening Test (DDST)-II 25

    Respiratory Distress Scoring 26

    Evaluate for Systemic Causes of Poor Weight Gain 29

    Check for Adequacy of Ventilator Settings.................................... 29

    Check for Adequacy of Bubble CPAP Settings 30

    Assessing Fontanel 30

    Hammersmith Neonatal Neurological Examination...................... 31

    New Ballard Score 33

Chapter 3. Emergency Assessment/Stabilization 40

    Identifying a Sick Newborn 35

    Assess for Jaundice Severity 36

    Respiratory Distress 37

    Shock... 39

    Hypoglycemia 40

    Seizures 41

    Abnormal Movements (not Seizures)...42

Assessing Hydration 43
Excessive Crying 45
Vomiting 46
Previous Sibling Unexpected Death 47
Cough in a Neonate 48
Case Studies: Jaundice 49
Case Studies: Respiratory Distress 53
Case Studies: Sick Newborn 56

Chapter 4. Case Studies 67
Cardiology 64
Electrolyte Disturbances 68
Infections in the Newborn 73
Musculoskeletal 78
Jaundice 82
Inborn Errors of Metabolism 89
Nutrition and Growth 94
Nephrology 97
Emergency and Critical Care 101
Necrotizing Enterocolitis 104
Adopted Baby 106
Gastroesophageal Reflux 107
Thyroid Disorders in the Newborn 110
Retinopathy of Prematurity Screening 113
Statistics 120

Chapter 5. Drugs 127
Adenosine 124
Adrenaline 125
Magnesium Sulfate 125
Erythromycin 125
Lyophilized Amphotericin 126
Amphotericin 127
Calcium Gluconate 128
Thiamine 128
Pyridoxine 128
Anti-D 128
Dextrose 129
Diazoxide 129
Milrinone 130
Fluconazole 132
Fosphenytoin 132
Intravenous Immunoglobulin (IVIG) 133
Linezolid 133
Low Molecular Weight Heparin 134
Nitric Oxide 135
Normal Saline 136
Dexamethasone 136
Betamethasone 137

Propranolol 138
Phenobarbitone 139
Probiotics 139
Sildenafil 140
Vancomycin 141
Alpostin 142

Chapter 6. Instruments 147
Bilirubinometer 143
FiO$_2$ monitor 144
Fluxmeter 144
Neonatal Incubator 145
Infusion Pump 146
Multichannel (Multi-parameter) Monitor 147
Phototherapy Unit 148
Pulse Oximeter 148
Radiant Warmer 149
Self-inflating Bag and Mask 150
Syringe Pump 151
Weighing Machine 152

Chapter 7. Imaging 158
Interpretation of Chest X-ray/Abdomen 153
Neonatal Cranial Ultrasound 171
Echocardiogram 176
Magnetic Resonance Imaging 179

Chapter 8. Interpretation 186
Arterial Blood Gas 186
Capnography 191
C-reactive Protein 192
Cardiotocography 193
Denver Developental Screening Test-II
Interpretation of Reports 197
Neonatal Electroencephalogram 200
Genetics 210
Intrauterine Growth Chart 219
Hepatobiliary Case Studies 220
Jaundice Evaluation 224
Microerythrocyte Sedimentation Rate 227
Neurology Case Studies 227
Partograph 232
Peripheral Smear 234
Pulse Oximeter Predischarge 239
Shake Test 240
Neonatal Surgery 241

Chapter 9. Observed Station 249
Neonatal Resuscitation 249
Phenobarbital Administration 251

Unexplained Birth Asphyxia 252
Counseling 253
Sudden Neonatal Death in Unit 254
Sudden Death of a Newborn in the Unit..............................255
Previous Sibling Unexpected Death 255
Consent for a New Drug or Trial 256
Consent for Therapeutic Hypothermia 257
Death of ELBW Baby 258
Death of a Baby after a Prolonged Hospital Stay 259
Death of Baby Operated for Diaphragmatic Hernia..............260

Chapter 10. Miscellaneous 262
India Demographics Spots...262
Spots..269

Index 281

1

Focused
History Taking

INSTRUCTIONS TO FACILITATOR

- Read aloud to the learner the following instructions and the case. Provide prompts where shown in italics (following the word "Prompt").
- As you observe the learner, note the assessment done or not done.
- Facilitator to speak:
  - "I am going to read a role play case. Please listen carefully, and then tell me what you would do to take care of this baby."
  - "I will not volunteer information unless you ask. I will provide no other feedback until the end of the case."

Overall Evaluation of the Learner

- Is polite, compassionate, uses gestures, speaks slowly and clearly, talks less and provokes informant more to speak.

At the Beginning the Learner Should

- Introduces self and greets the informant.
- Informs about what is going to be done.

At the End the Learner Should

- Asks the informant if there is any question or any query.
- Thanks the informant.

PRETERM ADMISSION AT BIRTH

Admission of Preterm Infant at Birth to NICU

1.	Chief complaints
2.	**Birth history** • Age in hours (date and time of birth) • Birth weight • Sex of the infant • Gestation

Contd...

Contd...

- Single or multiple pregnancy
- Hospital or home delivery
- Normal or cesarean section delivery
- Spontaneous, induced, precipitated or assisted delivery
- Problems during delivery
- Cry status or need for resuscitation
- Vitamin K status

3. **Maternal history**
   - Age
   - Para and gravida of the mother
   - Expected date of delivery
   - Blood group—Rh status
   - Consanguinity
   - No. of prenatal visits
   - Prenatal ultrasound details
   - Use of any medications
   - Previous complications of pregnancy
   - Prenatal steroids
   - Previous sibling status (age, well being, interventions in newborn period)

4. **Maternal risk factors**
   - Illness [(e.g. diabetes mellitus (DM), hypertension, asthma, etc.)]
   - Perinatal factors [(e.g. fetal distress, meconium liquor, oligo-polyhdramnios, fever, bleeding per vaginal, preterm premature rupture of membrane (PPROM), difficult labor, prolonged labor, multiple per vaginal examinations, uterine tenderness, foul liquor)]

5. **Family history**
   - Previous preterm delivery
   - Medical illness recurring in family [(e.g. congenital malformation, genetic disorder, DM, hypertension, asthma, allergy, heart disease, Kochs disease, deafness, kidney disease, sudden infant death syndrome (SIDS), thalassemia)]
   - Unexplained deaths in sibling or family members

6. **Social history**
   - Occupation
   - Parental educational status
   - Religion
   - Average monthly income
   - Smoking
   - Alcohol

FEEDING HISTORY TAKING

Assess for breastfeeding adequacy in a D7, 36 weeks infant who is not gaining weight

1.	Why does caregiver feel baby not gaining weight? Loose folds of skin? Weight? Subjective?
2.	Current weight compared to birth weight. Regained birth weight? By what day of life?

Contd...

Contd...

3. **Feeding history:**
   a. Type of feeds: Breast milk or formula or animal milk?
   b. No. of times/24 hours, night feeds
   c. If breastfed:
      i. Demand/scheduled feeding/switching breasts between feeds
      ii. Maternal breast or nipple problems such as sore nipples?
      iii. Method of feeding: Direct/paladai
   d. If formula/animal milk:
      i. Dilution
      ii. Method of feeding: Paladai/bottle
      iii. Type of formula
   e. Pattern of feeding: Does baby feed well/poorly (sick child)/frantic sucking (hyperthyroidism)/suck rest suck

4. **Adequacy of feeds:**
   a. Urine output:
      i. Number of wet diapers per day? (Indicator of hydration status and polyuria)
      ii. Color of urine (concentrated/smoky for urine infection/urate crystals)
   b. Stool pattern:
      i. Number of stools per day
      ii. Consistency of stools—normal semisolid/pellet like/ loose stools (adequacy of feeds/infection/malabsorption)
   c. Sleep: Duration of sleep after each feed

5. **Perinatal history:**
   a. Prenatal:
      – Maternal illnesses or infections TORCH [toxoplasmosis, other (syphilis, varicella-zoster, parvovirus B19), rubella cylomegalovirus and herpes] infection, hypertension (HTN), DM)]
      – Review of anomaly scan, intrauterine growth, liquor volume (polyhydramnios with Barter syndrome)
      – Maternal drug intake
   b. Natal
      – Preterm, or post-maturity, twins
      – Risk for asphyxia (e.g. fetal monitoring, liquor, meconium staining, Apgar's)
   c. Postnatal
      – Admission to intensive care unit (ICU), need for oxygen, blood transfusion, intravenous (IV) medications, surgery, total parenteral nutrition (TPN).
      – Results of newborn screening tests (e.g. congenital adrenal hyperplasia (CAH), galactosemia, thyroid stimulating hormone (TSH)
      – Maternal depression (medication review of drugs)
      – Recurrent infections (immunodeficiency)

6. **Family History:**
   • Consanguinity
   • Previous siblings with failure to thrive or other significant illness
   • F/H of poor weight gain (e.g. immunodeficiency, communicable disease like tuberculosis)

7. Asks the informant if there is any question or any query

4 INADEQUATE BREAST MILK

1.	Asks about onset time of the complaint
2.	Ask if the informant is able to breastfeed and if the answer is yes asks about duration of each feeding session. **OR** If the answer to the above question is "No" asks about the nature and quantity and frequency of top feeds.
3.	Tries to assess adequacy of breastfeeding to determine if it is only perceived breast milk insufficiency or actually inadequate breast milk production: Speaks that "Breast feeding is considered adequate if there is softening of breast after a feeding session and the neonate sleeps well between the breastfeeding sessions, passes urine at least 6–8 times in a day, crosses birth weight by 2 weeks and gains at least 25–30 g per day after the initial 7–10 days."
4.	Asks about the birth details and any labor interventions
5.	Asks about any maternal apprehensions (with regard to jaundice or any other concerns), stress or worry, history of medical or surgical illness or infertility, sub-optimal initiation of breastfeeding, early supplementation, maternal medication (including oral contraceptives; antihypertensives), any doubt any pain
6.	Asks about the time of initiation of the first breastfeed
7.	Asks about the separation of the infant from the mother
8.	Asks about the use of prelacteals, soothers or artificial feeding
9.	Asks about the over-stimulation by visitors and family, forcing the baby to breast
10.	Asks about prolonged breastfeeding attempts, inefficient latch or feeding and insufficient intake at breast or any pain in the breast
11.	Asks about previous experience of breastfeeding

RESPIRATORY DISTRESS

Day 1, near term, born to primi, vaginal delivery is brought with breathing difficulty over last few hours

1.	Time of onset (hours)
2.	Trend: Is respiratory distress (RD) same, improving or worsening
3.	What is the gestation?
4.	History of weak or absent cry at birth or need for resuscitation History of worsening on bag and mask resuscitation
5.	History of Prolonged labor, fetal distress, meconium stained liquor, difficult delivery
6.	History of assisted/precipitate delivery/Elective cesarean section
7.	History of maternal fever, foul smelling liquor, prolonged labor, multiple per vaginal examinations, PROM >12 hours, PPROM, assisted delivery
8.	History of antenatal steroids to mother, infant of diabetic mother (IDM), Rh isoimmunization

Contd...

Contd...

9.	History of polyhydramnios–oligohydramnios
10.	History of placenta previa or abruption
11.	Family history of unexplained neonatal deaths, stillbirths
12.	History of audible breathing sounds

SHOCK

Term, d3, 2.5 kg is brought with decreased feeding and decreased activity since last few hours

1.	**Feeding:** Breast or non-human milk fed? Frequency of feed, adequacy of feed
2.	**Asphyxia risk:** Prolonged labor, difficult labor, assisted delivery, fetal distress, meconium-stained liquor, need for resuscitation at birth
3.	**Sepsis risk:** Maternal fever, foul smelling liquor, prolonged labor, multiple per vaginal examinations, PROM >12 hours, assisted delivery, discharge from any site
4.	**Losses:** Vomiting, loose stools, umbilical ooze
5.	**Bleeding per vaginal**: Placenta previa or abruption
6.	Previous unexplained neonatal deaths
7.	Sudden unexplained deterioration
8.	Bleeding per oral/rectal or any site
9.	Abnormal movements of limbs, eyes or body
10.	Jaundice noted. Maternal infant blood group
11.	Abnormal odor to body or urine

HYPOGLYCEMIA

6 hours, term 1.9 kg, born to primi gravida mother, normal vaginal delivery is brought for poor activity and noted to have Glucostix of 25 mg% on admission

1.	Feeding pattern: Breast or non-human milk feed, frequency and adequacy of feeding
2.	Evaluation for sugar bedside since birth
3.	Maternal diabetes (controlled or poorly controlled)
4.	Intrapartum glucose infusion

Contd...

Contd...

5. Maternal drugs (e.g. β-blockers, terbutaline, oral hypoglycemic agents)

6 Intrapartum asphyxia (fetal distress, meconium liquor, need for resuscitation at birth, prolonged labor, difficult or assisted delivery)

7. Sepsis risk: Maternal fever, foul smelling liquor, prolonged labor, multiple per vaginal examinations, PROM > 12 hours, assisted delivery, discharge from any site

8. Abnormal movements of limbs, eyes or body

9. Abnormal odor to body or urine

10. Unexplained neonatal deaths

11. Previous sibling with hypoglycemia

JAUNDICE

Assess for Jaundice on Day 3

1. Asks about onset of jaundice (age <24 hours/>24 hours old age)

2. Extent of jaundice (skin, sclera, body part, palms-soles)

3. Feeding: Breast milk or formula or animal milk?

4. Current weight compared to birthweight.
   Does the neonate have excessive weight loss (the students calculates the weight loss in grams and percentage and interprets as normal or abnormal)

5. Assess breastfeeding adequacy by number of wet diapers per day

6. Infections (pustules, discharge from any site, feeding, etc.) or fever?

7. Asks about the intake of any medications in the newborn or mother

8. Asks and notes the gender and ethnicity?
   If relevant (males, kutch, parsis have some increased risk)

9. Asks the neonate and mothers blood group

10. Asks about feeding pattern (decreased, poor, inability to feed, regular)

11. Asks about cry (shrill, poor, lusty)

12. Asks about sensorium (alert, active, drowsy, irritable, lethargic)

13. Asks about abnormal movements

14. Asks about primi or no/abortion/preterm/intrauterine growth restriction (IUGR)/post maturity/twins

15. Asks maternal blood group (repeated)/if Rh –ve ask about anti-D

16. Asks maternal illnesses or infections (TORCH infection, HTN, DM)

17. Asks results of antenatal screening tests [human immunodeficiency virus (HIV)/hepatitis B surface antigen(HBsAg)]

18. Asks mode of delivery, instrument uses (birth trauma with bruising cephalohematoma)

19. Asks precipitate delivery (could indicate polycythemia)

Contd...

Contd...

20. Asks risk for asphyxia (e.g. fetal monitoring, liquor, meconium staining, Apgars)

21. Asks risk for sepsis (e.g. maternal fever, foul liquor, uterine tenderness, PROM >18 hours, PPROM, multiple per vaginal examinations, etc.)

22. Asks about any intervention (partial exchange/ double volume exchange, phototherapy, intravenous fluids, oxygen or neonatal intensive care unit (NICU) admission, fever, intravenous medications, surgery, TPN)

23. Asks results of newborn screening tests (e.g. galactosemia, TSH)

24. Asks about consanguinity

25. Asks about previous siblings with neonatal jaundice

26. Asks about other family members with jaundice, anemia or blood disorders, splenectomy, bile stones or gallbladder removal

27. Asks for history of phototherapy

2

Focused
Clinical Examination

WELL BABY EXAMINATION

General Examination of Newborn

Pattern of evaluation (order of examination may vary but all need to be covered):

1. **Observing the baby:** Consciousness, color, tone, posture, cry, activity (identifies stable, unstable, not well and in need of further assessment).
2. **Vitals:** Temperature, heart rate (HR), respiratory rate (RR), blood pressure (BP), pulse oximeter (baseline data, to look at trend, to identify well or not well).
3. Anthropometry and gestation.
4. Head-to-toe physical examination.
5. Occult congenital anomaly.
6. Danger signs.

Look	Normal	Abnormal
Consciousness	Alert	Drowsy, lethargic, nonresponsive, persistent irritability, asleep
Color	Pink	Pale (anemia, shock), plethora (polycythemia), dusky [cold stress, hypothermia, congenital heart disease (CHD), shock], cyanosis (cold stress, CHD, respiratory failure)
Tone, posture	Active with good tone and responds to pain	Abnormal tone is reflected by posture (frog legged posture, extended posture) and suggests neurologic compromise
Cry	Lusty cry	Weak, absent, ill sustained or shrill cry
Activity	Symmetric and spontaneous	Decreased, absent, asymmetric and abnormal movements.
Temperature	36.5–37.5°C	Cold stress (36–36.5°C), hypothermia (<36°C), core-axillary mismatch (>3°C) or fever (>37.5°C)

Contd...

Contd...

Look	Normal	Abnormal
Perfusion	Heart rate, color, core-axillary temperature, capillary refill time, urine output, blood pressure	To identify early shock. Monitor the trends. More the parameters abnormal, more is the possibility of shock. Fall in blood pressure (hypotension) is late sign of shock and is ominous sign
Breathing	Regular, rate 40–60/min, no audible sounds	Slow <40 or fast >60 per min, Downes score or Silverman Anderson score, apnea, gasping, chest indrawing, grunt, stridor
Pulse oximeter	>95% after 24 hours of age	UL and LL difference of >5, SpO_2 <90% in room air

Look	Rationale
Anthropometry	Weight, height and head circumference plotting on growth chart defines growth pattern
Gestation	Preterms (<34 weeks), post-terms, late preterm (34–37 weeks) are vulnerable population

Head-to-Toe Physical Examination

Assess	Look for	Abnormal
Skin	Hydration, color	Birthmarks, congenital anomaly
Head	Size, shape, symmetry Fontanel, sutures	Microcephaly and macrocephaly, molding, craniosynostosis, tense anterior fontanelle, swelling
Eyes	Size, position, slant	White reflex, asymmetry, discharge, redness
Ears	Shape, size, position	Low set, tags, pits, malformation
Mouth	Shape, position, symmetry	Tongue, gums, tooth, swelling
Palate	Anterior/posterior palate	Cleft
Limbs	Symmetry, movements, palmar crease	Polydactyly, syndactyly, clinodactyly, malformation
Genitalia	*Boys*: Penile size, urethral opening, scrotal symmetry, rugosity, testis in scrotum *Girls*: Labia majora-minora, clitoris, urethra-vagina	Penis <1 cm, chordee, hypospadias, epispadias, absent scrotal rugosity, empty scrotum, asymmetric scrotum Hymenal tags, discharge per urethra-vagina
Back—spine	Spine curvature	Defect, tufts of hair
Hips	Thigh crease symmetry, Barlows-Otolarni	Asymmetry, leg shortening

Contd...

Note	Comment
Occult congenital anomalies	Isolated cleft palate, cataract, anogenital anomalies, spinal defects and absent femorals need to be specifically looked at
Danger signs (Grunt, cyanosis, worsening, sensorium, apnea)	To identify life-threatening events and consider urgent transfer/interventions

BREASTFEEDING

Assessment for Breastfeeding

Examines the breast for flat nipple/inverted nipple/ engorgement/pain/sore nipples or mastitis in the breast after informing the informant

Examines the neonate for evidence of dehydration (assess for weight, sunken fontanel, pallor, lethargy and overall activity)

Examines a direct breastfeeding session and evaluates for cardinal points of positioning (Fig. 1):
• Head in line with the body
• Whole body well supported
• Neonate turned toward the mother
• Neonate's abdomen touching the mother's abdomen

Examines a direct breastfeeding session and evaluates for cardinal points of attachment (Figs 2A and B):
• More areola visible above the neonate's mouth than below it
• Neonate's mouth is wide open
• Neonate's lower lip is turn outward
• Neonate's chin is touching the mother's breast

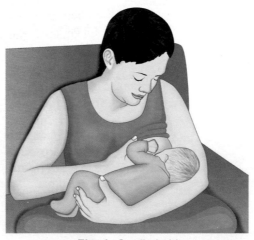

Fig. 1: Cradle hold

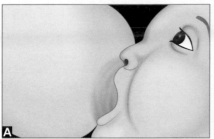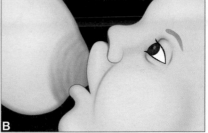

Figs 2A and B: (A) A baby well attached to his mother's breast; (B) A baby poorly attached to his mother's breast

WEIGHT, LENGTH AND OCCIPITOFRONTAL CIRCUMFERENCE (OFC) MEASUREMENT

Measurement of Length

Equipment: Infantometer, cloth for covering the base, mother or assistant.

Procedure

- Ask the assistant or mother to help with measurement and to comfort the baby
- Cover the length board with a thin cloth or soft paper
- Explain to the assistant where to stand when placing the baby on length board, i.e. opposite to you, on the side of the length board away from the tape
- Lay the baby on his back with his head against the fixed headboard, compressing the hair
- Position the head so that an imaginary vertical line from the ear canal to the lower border of the eye socket is perpendicular to the board (the baby's eyes should be looking straight up)
- Ask the assistant to hold the head in this position
- Check that the infant lies straight along the board and does not change position. Shoulders should touch the board, and the spine should not be arched
- Hold down the infant's legs with one hand and move the footboard with the other. Apply gentle pressure to the knees to straighten the legs as far as they can go without causing injury
- While holding the knees, pull the footboard against the infant's feet. The soles of the feet should be flat against the footboard, toes pointing upwards
- Read the measurement and record the infant's length in centimeters to the last **completed** 0.1 cm in the notes of the growth record. This is the last line that you can actually see (0.1 cm = 1 mm)

Note

- If an infant is extremely agitated and both legs cannot be held in position, measure with one leg in position

- If the infant bends the toes and prevents the footboard from touching the soles, scratch the soles slightly and slide in the footboard quickly when the infant straightens the toes
- Record the length on the growth chart and present as length in centiles (Figs 3A and B).

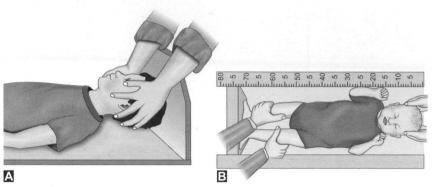

Figs 3A and B: Measurement of length

Measurement of Weight

Equipment: Digital weighing scale, accurate and has a precision of weighing 0.01 kg or 10 grams. Has an option of zeroing.

Procedure

Ask the mother or assistant to assist you in weighing the baby	
Ensure a sterile baby towel is placed on the pan	
Ensure zeroing of the machine before placing the baby	
Weight the baby naked	
Note the value once the baby is relatively calm. Wait for the fluctuations to settle down	
Record the weight on the growth chart and present as weight in centiles	

Measurement of the head circumference

Equipment: A flexible and non-stretchable tape

Procedure

Ask the mother to assist you by making the baby comfortable	
Position the tape just above the eyebrows, above the ears and around the biggest part of the back of the head	
Pull the tape snugly to compress the hair	
The overlapping of the tape should be done on the lateral aspect of the head (avoid the curves), to get accurate value	
Read the nearest 0.1 cm, by cross tape technique	
Plot the head circumference on the growth curve and present in centiles (Fig. 4)	

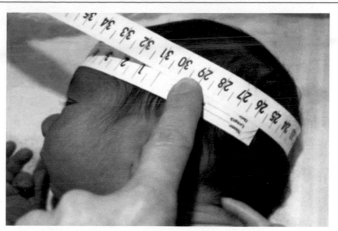

Fig. 4: Measurement of head circumference

CAPILLARY REFILL TIME

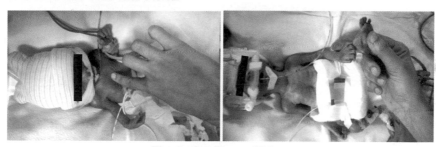

Fig. 5: Capillary refill time

Capillary refill time (CRT) is time taken for color to return to an external capillary bed after pressure is applied to cause blanching (Fig. 5)

Procedure

- Ensure warmth
- Expose the chest of the infant
- Use thumb or finger and press on the sternum for 5 seconds
- Remove the thumb/finger and see the time taken for blanched area to become pink again

Note

- The mnemonic used is "one in one thousand, two in one thousand, three in one thousand, four in one thousand, five in one thousand"
- The normal CRT is less than 3 seconds.

BLOOD PRESSURE MEASUREMENT BY OSCILLOMETRY

- Select the appropriate size of blood pressure cuff (too large gives falsely low BP readings and vice-versa)
- Clean the cuff with chlorhexidine based hand rub if the used cuff is reusable
- Place the cuff over the arm snugly fitting aligning with the course of the underlying artery
- Before taking a reading ensure the baby is in a quiet but alert state
- Take at least three reading few minutes apart
- Note the average reading
- Interpret the BP using gestation based centile BP charts and the clinical condition of the baby
- Remove the cuff from the arm

Note
- Preferably, use a separate cuff for each infant to prevent cross infection
- Length of the BP cuff bladder should be at least 80% of the distance of the upper arm from the point of the shoulder and the breadth of the BP cuff bladder should be at least 60% of the perimeter of the upper limb.

Cuff number (size)	Limb circumference
1	3–6 cm
2	4–8 cm
3	6–11 cm

- Avoid the conditions that can increase the BP like crying, feeding, pain, and turmoil.

DEVELOPMENTAL DYSPLASIA OF HIP

- Inspection and examination
  1. Exposure:
     a. Undress the baby to examine the spine and hip
  2. Perform general observation
     a. Grossly note general health status
     b. Look for dysmorphic features
        i. Teratological developmental dysplasia of hip accompanies arthrogryposis and spinal dysraphism
        ii. Inspect the back for spina bifida or meningocele.
     c. Look for associated disorders with DDH
        i. Plagiocephaly
        ii. Torticollis
        iii. Calcaneovalgus foot
        iv. Metatarsus adductus

3. Perform lower limb examination
   a. Inspect for limb length discrepancy (Galeazzi sign).
      i. Flex lower limbs at knees
      ii. Place heels together with soles of feet flat on bed
      iii. Make sure pelvis is square and look at level of knees
          Inequality in the height of the knees is a positive Galeazzi sign
   b. Inspect thigh creases, groin crease and gluteal folds by holding up the child as well as placing the child prone
      i. Any asymmetry on ventral/dorsal surfaces
4. Test abduction
   a. Flex hips to right angle and test range of abduction
   b. Dislocated hip will be tighter and have restriction of movement.
5. Specific test
   a. Barlow test: Provocative dislocation of a reduced hip
      i. It is positive when an enlocated (suggest unstable) hip can be dislocated or subluxated. Each hip should be examined separately. The pelvis should be stabilized by holding the contralateral hip.
         - Flex lower limb at knee and hip
         - Adduct the baby's hip, gently applying a downward force by pushing the knee gently posteriorly (i.e. downwards)
         - Normally, there is a small amount of movement
         - But in abnormal hip, the force will subluxate/dislocate the joint and a "clunk" will be felt
   b. Ortalani test: Reduction maneuver of a dislocated hip.
      i. It is positive when a dislocated hip is relocated
         - Place thumbs medially and index finger high on posterolateral aspect of thigh (behind greater trochanter)
         - Hips flexed to 90 degrees and gently abducted, simultaneously exerting upward pressure through the greater trochanter
         - Normally, smooth abduction
         - But in dislocated hip, the force will relocate the head in the acetabulum at the joint and a "clunk" will be felt
   c. Klisic's test:
      i. Line drawn from greater trochanter to anterior superior iliac spine (ASIS) should continue medially
      ii. If line pass towards the umbilicus—hip is normal
      iii. If line passes below umbilicus—hip is dislocated
- Dress child
- Thank parent/examiner
- Wash hands.

Task: Assess Risk Factors for Developmental Dysplasia of Hip

- Female child
- Family history
- First coming part (Breech presentation)
- First born
- Fluid (oligohydraminos)
- Feet deformity
- Fetal anomalies.

JAUNDICE

Perform a Focused Examination for this Newborn with Jaundice

Focused clinical assessment	
Assess	Rationale
Gestation (based on physical and neurological criterion)	Preterm, near term is increased risk for significant jaundice
Vital parameters (temperature, RR, HR, SpO$_2$)	Sick babies (unstable vital parameters, change in activity, sleep or feeding) are more at risk for severe jaundice and bilirubin encephalopathy
Weight (check weight/ dehydration)	Weight loss at discharge >3% per day or >7% cumulative weight loss is suggestive of inadequate feeds which is a contributory factor for significant jaundice. SGA, LGA are more at risk for jaundice. SGA status may be secondary to intrauterine infection
Age in hours—history	Hour-specific bilirubin nomogram can predict babies likely to develop significant jaundice. The decision making is based on interpretation of total serum bilirubin (TSB) in relation to age in hours. Visible jaundice in first 24 hours is always pathological. A jaundice beyond 14 days merits investigations Ask or look for fever, vomiting, convulsions, distress, lethargy, abdominal distention, bleeding tendency, or jitteriness
Extent of jaundice	Jaundice staining the palms and soles is severe jaundice. Not reliable in preterm, under phototherapy and in dark pigmented babies
Urine/stool pattern	High-colored urine and clay stools suggests direct hyperbilirubinemia. Frequent passage of urine which is colorless assures adequacy of feeding
Plethora	Flushed appearance suggests plethora. Polycythemia independently aggravates jaundice due to high RBC turnover
Pallor, hepatomegaly or splenomegaly	Suggests hemolytic jaundice/IU infection/ sepsis and high risk for developing severe hyperbilirubinemia
Petechiae	Symptoms of sepsis, IU infection, erythroblastosis
Signs of sepsis	Assess for activity, pustules, umbilical discharge, temperature fluctuation, foul smell, rash, signs of poor perfusion

Contd...

Contd...

Assess	Rationale
Microcephaly	Suggests intrauterine infection
Bruises, cephalhematoma	Aggravates jaundice
Activity, feeding	Decreased activity, sleepy and not feeding well on the breast needs evaluation of underlying cause and bilirubin encephalopathy
Dysmorphism	Trisomy, syndromes
Midline defects	Suggestive of hypopituitarism
Fundus/cataract	Chorioretinitis, Suggestive of IU infection
Neonatal reflexes (suck, Moro's reflex, asymmetric tonic neck reflex, grasp)	Asymmetry, partial, absent is pathological and suggests bilirubin encephalopathy

Abbreviations: RR, respiratory rate; HR, heart rate; LGA, large for gestational age; SGA, small for gestational age; RBC, red blood cells; IU, intrauterine

Summarize

- Well or sick
- Term or preterm
- Age in hours
- Extent of jaundice
- Positive physical finding
- Hydration status
- Symptoms of indirect/direct jaundice
- With or without bilirubin encephalopathy.

MORO EXAMINATION

Ensure the baby is alert and in quiet state

Ensure head is in midline

Head drop method: The infant is held suspended in a symmetrical supine position with one of the examiner's hands behind the chest and the other supporting the head, allow the head to be dropped back a few cm

Note
a. Abduction of the upper limbs (spreading out arms)
b. Adduction of the upper limbs (unspreading the arms)
c. Opening of the fist
d. Crying
e. The reflex is complete and symmetrical on both the sides

Note

- This primitive reflex emerges at 8–9 weeks in utero, is present at birth and normally disappears after 3 or 4 months
- An absent reflex is seen in upper motor neuron lesions, e.g. severe perinatal asphyxia, intracranial hemorrhage, infection, brain malformation, general muscular weakness of any cause, and cerebral palsy (CP) of the spastic type

- An asymmetric Moro is most often seen with local cause, e.g. damage to peripheral nerve (brachial plexus lesion, cervical cord lesion) or fracture bone (clavicle)
- Postnatal persistence occurs in infants with severe neurological defects
- An exaggerated response may also be detected in infants with a severe bilateral intrauterine lesion (e.g. hydranencephaly)
- Ensure that both the subject's hands are open at the moment of elicitation of the reflex so as not to provoke an asymmetrical response
- If the baby is crying, allow the baby to quiet down.

POPLITEAL ANGLE

Assess the Tone of the Hamstring Muscles

Ensure the newborn is in quiet and alert state
Elicit on one leg at a time
Ensure that the pelvis is not lifted off the bed
With the infant lying supine, remove the diaper
The thigh is placed gently on the baby's abdomen with the knee fully flexed. Wait until the infant stops kicking actively before extending the leg
Gently grasp the foot at the sides with one hand while supporting the side of the thigh with the other. Extend the leg until a definite resistance to extension is appreciated
Note the angle between the thigh and the leg. It is typically about 90 degrees
Compare response of both the legs

Note

- Extension of the leg beyond 90–120° would be seen in hypotonia
- The prenatal frank breech position will interfere with this maneuver for the first 24–48 hours (Fig. 6).

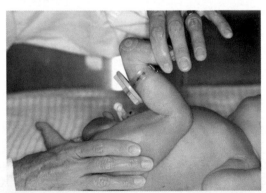

Fig. 6: Popliteal angle measuring

HEEL TO EAR EXAMINATION

Procedure

Ensure the infant is quiet

The infant is placed supine

Support the infant's thigh laterally alongside the body with the palm of one hand. The other hand grasps the infant's foot at the sides to pull it toward the ipsilateral ear

Note the location of the heel where significant resistance is appreciated. Observe the distance between feet and head

Keep the pelvis flat on the bed

Elicit on one leg at a time

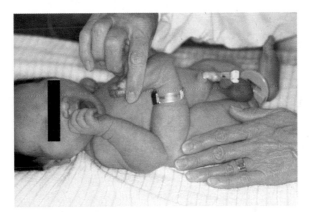

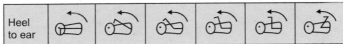

Fig. 7: Heel to ear examination

Note

- The heel in a normal baby would only come to mid chest. If the foot can be drawn to the ear then there is hypotonia (Fig. 7).

SCARF SIGN

Procedure

- Ensure the infant is in supine position, alert but in a quiet state
- Hold the infant's hand and try to bring it around the neck and as posteriorly as possible over the opposite shoulder
- The other hand supports the baby's chest and the thumb of is placed on the infant's elbow
- The point on the chest to which the elbow moves easily prior to significant resistance is noted (Fig. 8)

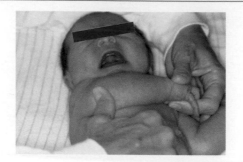

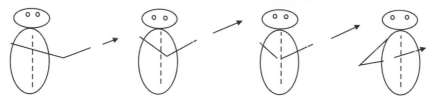

Fig. 8: Scarf sign

Note

- The hand should not go past the shoulder and the elbow should not cross the midline in term infants.

ASSESSMENT OF SHOULDER TONE

Focused Clinical examination

1. How to assess shoulder tone in newborn?

The assessment of shoulder tone in newborns includes:
a. **Posture**.
b. **Passive tone:** Ensure head in midline for all maneuvers to avoid effect of atonic neck reflex (ATNR).
c. Scarf sign.
d. Forearm recoil.
e. **Active tone:** Raise to sit and back to lying maneuver.
f. **Horizontal suspension**.
g. **Vertical suspension**.
h. **Primitive reflexes:** Finger grasp and response to traction.

2. Normal parameters for shoulder tone evaluation

Finding	<32 weeks	34 weeks	36 weeks	Term
Scarf sign				
Forearm recoil				
Raise to sit				
Back to lying				

Answer

Finding	<32 weeks	34 weeks	36 weeks	Normal term
Scarf sign	Arm encircles neck at 28 weeks	Elbow largely passes midline	Elbow slightly passes midline	Elbow does not cross midline
Forearm recoil	Extension	Weak	Present	Strong
Raise to sit	No head movement forwards	Head rolls on shoulder	Head briskly passes in axis	Perfect minimal lag
Back to lying	No head movement backwards	Head passes briskly in axis	Powerful movement backwards	Perfect minimum lag

3. Raise to sit and back to lying maneuver (Fig. 9).

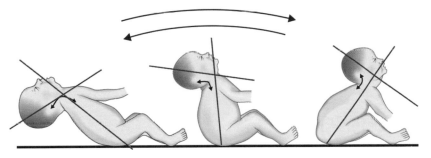

Fig. 9: Assessment of shoulder tone

Questions
a. Interpret the above result in a term neonate.
b. How would be the posture this baby when it is supine?

Answers
a. **Hypertonia of neck extensors**: Raise to sit—head does not pass the axis nor move forward at end of maneuver. Back to lying—movement is too good.
b. **Retrocollis**: Neck extended, head to one side

or

Opisthotonus: Arching of whole body axis with neck and spine extensor hypertonia.

4. What would you to look for in the general examination of a newborn baby with abnormal shoulder tone evaluation in each of the following?
a. Eyes.
b. Skin.
c. Head.
d. Face.
e. Mouth.
f. Chest.

g. Joints.

h. Spine.

Answers

a. **Eyes**: Hypertonia elevator palpebrae superioris, nystagmus, fix and track, acoustic blink.

b. **Skin:** Neurocutaneous markers.

c. **Head**: Anterior fontanels, sutures—overriding, squamous suture.

d. **Face:** Dysmorphic features (Downs, Prader Wili).

e. **Examination of mouth and tongue**:

   a. Palate—high arched (abnormal motor function of fetal tongue).

   b. Fasciculations at rest in periphery of tongue (Werdning Hoffmans).

f. **Chest movements:** Indrawing of sternum (Werdning Hoffman).

g. **Joints:** Arthogryposis (suggests antenatal neuromuscular etiology).

h. **Spine:** Dysraphism.

5. **What is the clinical significance of abnormal shoulder tone?**

The clinical significance of abnormal shoulder tone includes:

a. Also associated with trunk and neck abnormalities.

b. Increased or decreased shoulder tone delays midline hand play, reach and transfer.

c. Increased shoulder tone interferes with hand to mouth pattern.

PALMAR GRASP REFLEX

Ensure the infant is awake and alert
Ensure baby is lying in supine position on a flat comfortable surface/mother's lap with head in midline
Ensure that dorsum of hands (of baby) are not touching the bed/towel or any other object
Place little finger (preferably)/index finger along ulnar aspect of baby's palm and applies pressure gently onto palm
Note for appropriate response: Flexion of all fingers around the examiner's finger and closure of hand
Apply mild traction as if trying to pull finger away from baby's palm
Note for increasing tightening of baby's grip and clinging, one may also be able to gently lift a term baby off the couch with this grip itself
Gently remove the finger from baby's grip—if not able to remove, can gently stimulate the dorsum of same hand (which should elicit opening of hands)
Repeat the same process on the other side

Summarizes (when asked)

- Term/preterm
- Postmenstrual age/corrected age
- State or sensorium of baby
- Response—optimal/not optimal, symmetric/asymmetric.

Note

- Age of appearance: noted in utero around 16 weeks, may be elicited in a preterm by 25 weeks PMA
- Age of disappearance: Easily elicited in the first 3 months of life (corrected age if preterm), usually disappears by 6 months. Replaced by voluntary hand movements
- Note whether there are any attachments on the hands (SpO_2 probe, intravenous cannula) that can interfere with/affect response.

What is an abnormal response?

- If the reflex is not elicited/weak during the age when it normally should be present:
  - Usually lower motor neuron lesions like root, plexus, nerve, spinal cord injury
  - Generalized neonatal encephalopathy
  - May not be elicited in evolving athetoid cerebral palsy.
- If the reflex is exaggerated or persists beyond the age of normal disappearance: Spastic cerebral palsy
- Persistence may lead to poor handwriting, poor manual dexterity/fine motor skills (Fig. 10).

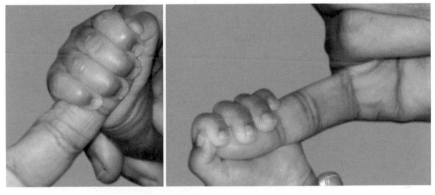

Fig. 10: Palmar grasp reflex

PLANTAR GRASP REFLEX

Ensure the baby is awake and alert

Ensure baby is lying in supine position on flat surface with head in midline

Place thumb on the sole of the foot below the toes and apply gentle pressure

Note appropriate response—flexion of all toes

Repeat on other side

Summarizes (when asked)

- Term/preterm
- Postmenstrual age/corrected age
- State or sensorium of baby
- Response—optimal/not optimal, symmetric/asymmetric.

Need to know
- Age of appearance: Elicited in preterm from 25 weeks postmenstrual age (PMA)
- Age of disappearance: Easily elicited in the first 6 months of life (corrected age if preterm), usually disappears by 12 months. Disappearance is significantly related to commencement of standing
- Notes whether there are any attachments on the feet (SpO$_2$ probe, intravenous cannula) that can interfere with/ affect response.

What is an abnormal response?

If the reflex is not elicited/weak during the age when it normally should be present:
- Usually lower motor neuron lesions like root, plexus, nerve, and spinal cord injury
- Generalized neonatal encephalopathy
- May not be elicited in evolving spastic cerebral palsy.

A weak or reduced plantar response has been shown to be a sensitive indicator of later development of spasticity. The side of abnormal response correlates well with the laterality of later motor abnormalities like in spastic hemiplegia.

If the reflex is exaggerated or persists beyond the age of normal disappearance: Athetoid cerebral palsy.

Persistence may lead to awkwardness while walking, poor balance and problems with sports requiring balance and coordination while running (Fig. 11).

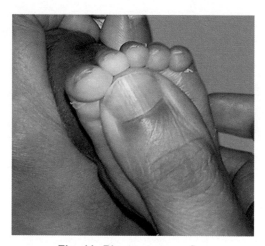

Fig. 11: Plantar grasp reflex

ASYMMETRIC TONIC NECK REFLEX

Ensure the baby is in a quiet but alert state
Ensures baby is in supine with head in midline to start with
Turn the head of the baby gently so that the face looks towards any one side
Note the appropriate response: The arms and legs on the side the face extend; and the other side limbs flex (classical fencing posture)
Repeat by turning the head to another side and note the response

Note

- Ensure there are no attachments on the hands (SpO_2 probe, intravenous cannula) that can interfere with/affect response
- If baby turns head spontaneously to any side—can note for appropriate response without touching the baby
- Age of appearance: 18 weeks of gestation (noted in utero)
- Age of disappearance: The reflex should be inhibited 4–6 months of age (corrected age if preterm) in the awake state, beyond which persistence is considered abnormal.

Differentials for Nonoptimal Response

- Decreased/no response can be normal (the reflex is best observed rather than elicited)
- Depressed sensorium due to various conditions leading to neonatal encephalopathy can lead to decreased response.

Asymmetric tonic neck reflex (ATNR) is required in early infancy to establish visual-motor (hand eye) coordination.

A retained ATNR is associated with abnormalities in motor, academic and social development domains. Infants and children are noted to have:

- Poor gross motor coordination and balance. Turning to any side might lead to change in ipsilateral limb tone and loss of balance
- Difficulty with visual tracking, activities that need crossing the midline like writing across a page from left to right or reading a line and following text
- Poor eye-hand coordination as in school learning and sports.

DENVER DEVELOPMENTAL SCREENING TEST (DDST)-II

1. What is the initial preparation necessary before administering the DDST-II?

Answer:

- Ensures environment is child friendly
- Child is well
- DDST-II kit and form available, kept ready out of sight of child
- Calculate corrected age
- Draw age line on chart
- Allay parental anxiety and reassure.

2. How to administer the DDST-II?

Answer:

- Do in presence of parents/caregiver
- Start administering items to the left of the line in the chart in each sector and continue to the right
- Administer items needing less active participation first like report, personal social, then fine motor-adaptive, language and lastly gross motor items

- In each sector, administer at least 3 items to the left of the line and every item intersected by the age line
- Testing may be flexible
- Rate test behavior after completion of the test
- Fill chart
- Explain results to parents and action plan.

3. Fill the table to interpret the result of development on a DDST-II chart?

Classification	Scores	Action
Normal		
Suspect		
Untestable		

Answer

Classification	Scores	Action
Normal	No delay +/– maximum 1 caution	Routine follow up
Suspect	2 or more caution and 1 or more delay	• Rescreen in 1–2 weeks • If retest suspect do DASII and neuromotor evaluation • Start early intervention
Untestable	Refusal in 1 or more item to left of line or refusal in 1 item in line in shaded area	• Rescreen in 1–2 weeks • If retest untestable or suspect do DASII and neuromotor evaluation • Start early intervention

RESPIRATORY DISTRESS SCORING

Case 1

A preterm male neonate with birth weight of 1,400 g and 30 weeks of gestation is born to primi gravida mother by cesarean section (Indication: Severe preeclampsia). The mother received complete course of antenatal steroids and magnesium sulfate before delivery. The infant has Apgar score of 7/8/8 at 1, 5 and 10 minutes, respectively. The infant developed respiratory distress immediately after birth and was started on T-Piece with blended oxygen. The infant was shifted to nursery the vitals of the infant were:

- Heart rate 148 beats/min
- Respiratory rate 68/min
- Audible grunting without stethoscope
- Cyanosis on FiO_2 40%
- Barely audible bilateral air entry
- Upper chest having respiratory lag
- Minimal lower chest retraction

- Minimal xiphoid retraction
- Marked nasal flaring.

Questions

1. Which scoring system to be used to assess severity of respiratory distress?
2. What is the severity score of respiratory distress?
3. Can we use Silverman Andersen score (SAS) for term infants?
4. What is the importance of severity score in management of infant?

Answers

1. As the index infant is premature baby we will use Silverman Andersen score because:
   - Tells better about the functional residual capacity (FRC) of lung in case of respiratory distress syndrome (RDS)
   - Assessing decrease in air entry (component of Downe's score) in premature infants is difficult as they have very small chest.
2. The SAS score of this infant is 7/10. The various component of the scoring system is:

Features	0	1	2	Index case
Upper chest movements	None	Respiratory lag	Seesaw respiration	1
Lower chest retractions	None	Minimal	Marked	1
Xiphoid retractions	None	Minimal	Marked	1
Nasal flaring	None	Minimal	Marked	2
Grunting	None	Audible with stethoscope	Audible without stethoscope	2

Examine the infant from side of the warmer and draw an imaginary mid-axillary line and the chest anterior to the line is upper chest and below the line is lower chest. Always use the stethoscope for auscultation of grunting if there is no audible grunting.

3. Silverman Andersen score can be used both in preterm and term infants but it is better to avoid using Downe's Score in preterm infants.
4. The importance of severity score in management is:
   - Useful as a criteria for initiation of respiratory support (noninvasive) in newborns at a score of ≥3
   - SAS score ≥7 is indication of impending respiratory failure and shows needs for invasive ventilation
   - Objective way to assess the severity of respiratory distress
   - Monitoring of score at regular intervals tells us about improvement or deterioration of the respiratory distress.

Case 2

A term female infant is born with birth weight of 3240 g and 39 weeks of gestation to a primi gravida mother by cesarean section (Indication: Fetal distress with meconium-stained amniotic fluid).

The infant is vigorous and is given an Apgar score of 8/9/9 at 1, 5 and 10 minutes respectively. The infant developed respiratory distress immediately after birth and was started on T-Piece with blended oxygen keeping targeted saturation as goal. The infant was shifted to nursery and the vitals of the infant were:

- Heart rate 156 beats/min
- Respiratory rate 74/min
- Capillary refill time <3 second
- Audible grunting with stethoscope
- Cyanosis on FiO_2 50%
- Barely audible bilateral air entry
- Upper chest having respiratory lag
- Minimal lower chest retraction
- Minimal xiphoid retraction
- Marked nasal flaring.

Questions

1. Which scoring system to be used to assess severity of respiratory distress?
2. What is the severity score of respiratory distress?

Answers

1. We can use both SAS or Downe's score for assessment of severity of respiratory distress in this case. In term infants Downe's score is preferred as it tells about the oxygen requirement by the infant, hence telling severity of parenchymal disease.
2. The SAS score of the infant is 7. The Downe's score of the infant is 8. The various components of Downe's score are:

Features	0	1	2	Index case
Cyanosis	None	In room air	In 40% FiO_2	2
Retractions	None	Mild	Severe	1
Air entry	Normal	Decreased	Barely audible	2
Grunting	None	Audible with stethoscope	Audible without stethoscope	2
Respiratory rates (per minute)	<60	60–80	>80 or apnea	1

Downe's ≥7 is indication of impending respiratory failure and shows needs for invasive ventilation.

Note

- If infant is on invasive ventilation the maximum score of each scoring system will be 8 as these infants will not be having grunting, as glottis remains open because of endotracheal tube
- If infant is on continuous positive airway pressure (CPAP), the maximum SAS score will be 8 as it is not possible to see nasal flaring in these infants.

EVALUATE FOR SYSTEMIC CAUSES OF POOR WEIGHT GAIN

Temperature: Cold peripheries (Persistent cold stress), core periphery mismatch (>3°C: Sepsis)

Jaundice: High-colored urine, clay stools, jaundice >14 days

Skin: Bleeding from any site, rash, discharge from any site, discoloration

Infections: Look for pustules, discharge from any site, feeding, crying during micturition, etc. or fever

Respiratory system: Breathing difficulty, increased work of breathing, color change

Cardiovascular system: Color change, breathing difficulty, suck swallow pattern, sweating over forehead, bluish discoloration on crying

Central nervous system: Activity, sensorium (active, alert, drowsy, irritable, lethargic), cry (shrill, poor, lusty), abnormal movements

Gastrointestinal tract: Vomiting, regurgitation, arching of back, excessive irritability, abdominal distension

Polyuric state (e.g. diabetes insipidus, Bartter syndrome, etc.)

CHECK FOR ADEQUACY OF VENTILATOR SETTINGS

Settings	Adequacy or optimization
Peak inspiratory pressure or delta pressure	• Chest rise adequate (gentle rise of chest), air entry good • TV between 4 and 6 mL/kg • $PaCO_2$ between 40 and 50 mm of Hg
Positive end-expiratory pressure	• Minimal or no recessions • Adequate lung inflation on chest X-ray (6–8 posterior spaces) • Satuations between 90 and 95% • PaO_2 between 50 and 70 mm of Hg
FiO_2	• Satuations between 90 to 95% • PaO_2 between 50 and 70 mm of Hg
Rate	• Each breath of the infant is triggered
Ti	• On the flow time graph, there is some gap between inspiratory and expiratory flow
Flow	• The delivered peak inspiratory pressure (PIP) is as much as the set PIP • Inpiratory flow is greater than expiratory flow
Humidification	• Servo-controlled humidifier in invasive mode • Temperature displayed is 37°C • Heat wire in the inspiratory limb is present • No condensation in inspiratory limb • Some condensate in the expiratory limb

CHECK FOR ADEQUACY OF BUBBLE CPAP SETTINGS

Settings	Adequacy or optimization
Clinical adequacy	Comfortable baby. Regular respiration. No chest indrawing or grunt. Breath sounds bilaterally equal.
Continuous positive airway pressure	• Water is optimum in the bubble chamber • Bubbling sounds heart in the axilla on both sides • Satuations between 90 and 95% • PaO_2 between 50 and 70 mm of Hg • Adequate lung inflation on chest X-ray (6–8 posterior end of the ribs)
FiO_2	• Satuations between 90 and 95% • PaO_2 between 50 and 70 mm of Hg
Flow	• Bubbling is present in the bubble chamber and is continuous
Prongs	• Snuggly fit • No erythema or blanching on the alae nasi • There is a gap between the prongs and columella • Prongs fixed to cap and cap is covering the ears • Cap is fixed snuggly to the head
Humidification	• Servo-controlled humidifier in invasive mode • Temperature displayed is 37°C • Heat wire in the inspiratory limb is present • No condensation in inspiratory limb • Some condensate in the expiratory limb

ASSESSING FONTANEL

Ensure the baby is in supine position in quiet state.

Lift the head slightly from the bed

Palpate the anterior fontanel (AF) at the junction of coronal and sagittal suture

Note:
1. Pulsatility: Normal fontanel is pulsatile. Absence of pulsations suggest raised intracranial pressure
2. Size: Note the maximum anteroposterior diameter (AP) and transverse diameter (T) to calcucate the fontanel size = (AP + T)/2.
3. Contour: Normally the fontanel is at soft, level and flat. A bulging or sunken fontanel is abnormal
4. Auscultate for bruit. It is heard with atriovenous (AV) malformation

Palpate the posterior fontanel (PF) at the junction of lambdoidal and sagittal suture.

Comments

• Anterior fontanel closes between 4 and 26 months (median 13.8 months). The size of anterior fontanel ranges from 3 and 6 cm.
• Early closure of AF is seen with microcephaly or craniosynostosis. Large fontanel or delayed closure is seen with raised intracranial pressure, rickets, achondroplasia trisomy 21 and congenital hypothyroidism.
• Bulging fontanel is seen with crying, coughing or vomiting or increased

intracranial pressure (e.g. intracranial hemorrhage, meningitis, hydrocephalus, hypoxic ischemic injury). Sunken fontanel is seen with dehydration.

- The posterior fontanel closes by 2 months. The size ranges from 1 to 1.5 cm.

HAMMERSMITH NEONATAL NEUROLOGICAL EXAMINATION

1. Introduces to the family the purpose of testing

- Your baby has successfully overcome so many medical challenges with support from you and your family. It is important now, to ensure good future development by assessing the functioning of eyes, ears, and nervous systems.
- **Hammersmith neonatal neurological examination (HNNE) is a comprehensive evaluation of functioning of the nervous system.** Any deviation from "optimal", i.e. from what is common to babies, will need further evaluation and will help your baby.

2. Knows the right age to test the baby

- Gestation: HNNE is best tested at 2 weeks of age in term babies and estimated term age (40 weeks PMA) in preterm babies
- Baby should be awake and alert, not hungry and crying
- Center the baby's head—ask mother to hold gently.

3. Testing

- Optimal—noted in up to 90% of healthy newborns
- Suboptimal—found in <10% babies
- Single, transient signs have no clinical relevance. Persistence of signs over time and deviation from optimal in 2 or more signs warrant detail evaluation. The neurological evaluation is performed under the following heads.

  A. **Observe tone and posture—candidate may be asked to demonstrate any of the following:**

  a. Posture of baby in alert resting state—greater importance given to match the *lower limb posture* with picture on the chart. Watch for asymmetry in tone and posture (head should be in midline).

  b. Upper limb – traction—hold the wrist and *not the palm*, look and feel *tone at elbow*

  c. Upper limb—arm recoil.

  d. Lower limb traction—hold the ankle and *not the foot*, look and feel *tone at knee.*

  e. Popliteal angle—baby on bed, flex the thighs on to the abdomen, pelvis in contact with bed. Use index fingers to deflex the knee (popliteal) joint. Measure angle between leg and bed. Ensure head in midline before inferring asymmetry. Popliteal angle tightness is best interpreted in relation to leg traction (tone patterns—item i).

  f. Trunk in ventral suspension – look for trunk tone and limb tone.

  g. Head lag in pull to sit.

h. Head control—flexors and extensors—place the baby is sitting posture, encircle the chest with your palm and fingers. Allow the head to fall forwards gently (to test extensors) and watch for head being lifted transiently to straight position. Repeat the test with head allowed to fall backwards gently (to test flexors). Best evaluated by comparing the flexors and extensors (tone patterns—item i). Well-developed extensors in relation to flexors points to possibly evolving cerebral palsy.

i. Evaluate tone patterns—real difference in tone inferred if one column difference is found between compared items:
   - Upper—lower limb.
   - Popliteal—leg traction.
   - Head control flexor—extensor.

B. Movements
   a. Quantity and quality: Abnormal writhing, cramped, and stereotyped movements
   b. Abnormal movements: Tremors, startle, spontaneous abnormal movements that are persistent.

C. Abnormal patterns
   a. Cortical thumb, thumb, and index finger opposed.
   b. Spontaneous upgoing big toe, flexed toes of foot.

D. Reflexes
   a. Moro's—asymmetry in tone may suggest Erb's palsy or trauma. Depressed Moro's may be seen in HIE
   b. Palmar grasp
   c. Plantar grasp
   d. Sucking reflex
   e. Deep tendon reflexes
   f. Stepping and placing

E. Orientation
   a. Arousability and consolability—baby's change in behavior is noted as examiner uncovers the baby. Most babies will be easy to arouse and start crying (baby will appear difficult to arouse if baby just had a feed). If baby is difficult to calm by patting gently or cuddling, this may suggest abnormal behavior (baby will appear difficult to console if baby is hungry).
   b. Visual orientation—slowly dangling red ball or ring, or human face is presented at a distance about 18 inches (distance from breast to mother's face when baby is breastfed).
   c. Auditory orientation—sound introduced from behind (not in line of vision)—distance about 10-15 cm from ear (distance from breast to mother's face when baby is breastfed).

F. Examine head size, shape, and spine

4. Summarizes examination findings—interpretation
   a. As a screening tool—the suboptimal neuroposture or behavior are in "black" boxes, they need to be re-evaluated for persistence of signs.
   b. As a research tool—each evaluated item can be converted into scores. If 90% babies demonstrate the sign, it is considered as optimal. Items are scored as suboptimal or not optimal if only 10% or less of babies demonstrate the sign.

Practice Pointers

Strengths of HNNE

a. Comprehensive examination of all domains of nervous system.
b. Easy to do, even for non-neurologist.
c. Takes only 10–15 minutes to complete.
d. Good inter-observer reliability.
e. Allows evaluation for persistence of signs sand evolution of signs.
f. Validated against magnetic resonance imaging (MRI) in prediction of outcomes.

When is HNNE inaccurate?

a. Baby on sedatives or anti-epileptic drugs.
b. Isolated deviant signs have limited value. Deviation of one/two signs is found in one-third of the healthy population.

NEW BALLARD SCORE

Ask the learner to assess the gestation of a preterm baby by New Ballard Score (NBS) (Fig. 1). Baby should be preterm and gestation should be 28–34 weeks. Baby should be hemodynamically stable and age should be less than 96 hours (or less desirably <7days). Provide following chart and assess how gestation is assessed.

1. Performs hand hygiene
2. Examines as per chart (12 points)
   a. Completes all points
   b. Assesses each parameter by correct method
3. Provides value of assessed gestation.

Neuromuscular maturity

Score	-1	0	1	2	3	4	5
Posture							
Square window (wrist)	>90°	90°	60°	45°	30°	0°	
Arm recoil		180°	140°–180°	110°–140°	90°–110°	<90°	
Popliteal angle	180°	160°	140°	120°	100°	90°	<90°
Scarf sign							
Heel to ear							

Contd...

Contd...

Physical maturity

Skin	Sticky, friable, transparent	Gelatinous, red translucent	Smooth, pink; visible veins	Superficial peeling and/ or rash; few veins	Cracking, pale areas; rare veins	Parchment, deep cracking; no vessels	Leathery, cracked wrinided		
Lanugo	None	Sparse	Abundant	Thinning	Bald areas	Mostly baid	Maturity rating		
Plantar surface	Heel-100 40-50 mm: −1 <40 mm: -2	>50 mm, no crease	Faint red marks	Anterior transverse crease only	Crease anterior 2/3	Creases over entire sole	Score	Weeks	
							-10	20	
							-5	22	
Breast	Imperceptible	Barely percaptible	Flat arecla, no bud	Stippled areola, 1–2 mm bud	Raised areola, 3–4 mm bud	Full areola, 5–10 mm bud	0	24	
							5	26	
							10	28	
Eye/Ear	Lids fused loosely:-1 tightly:-2	Lids open; pinna flat; stays folded	Slightly curved pinna; soft slow recoil	Well curved pinna; soft but ready recoli	Raised areola, 30–4 mm bud	Testes pendulous, deep rugae	15	30	
							20	32	
							25	34	
Genitals (male)	Scrotum flat, smooth	Scrotum empty, faint, rugae	Testes in upper canal, rare rugae	Testes descending, few rugae	Testes down good rugae	Testes pendulous deep rugae	30	36	
							35	38	
							40	40	
Genitals (female)	Clitoris prominent, labia flat	Clitoris prominent, small labia minora	Clitoris prominent, enlarging minora	Majora and minora equally prominent	Majora large, minora small	Majora cover clitoris and minora	45	42	
							50	44	

Fig. 1

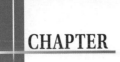

Emergency Assessment/ Stabilization

IDENTIFYING A SICK NEWBORN

Rapid Assessment to Identify if the Newborn is Well or Unwell

Look	Well	Unwell
Temperature	36.5–37.5°C	Cold stress, hypothermia, core-axillary mismatch or fever
Appearance	Alert	Drowsy, lethargic, nonresponsive, persistent irritability, abnormal movements, ear discharge
Breathing	Rate 40–60/min, regular, no audible sounds	Rate <40 or >60 per min, apnea, gasping, chest indrawing, grunt, stridor
Color	Pink	Pallor, plethora, icterus, cyanosis
Pulse oximeter	>95% after 24 hours of age	UL and LL difference of >5, SpO_2 <90%
Rationale	No active intervention	Hospitalize, stabilize, identify the cause, treat the cause

All unwell babies need detail evaluation, work up and treatment of the underlying cause.

Identify "Why" the Newborn is "at Risk" or "Unwell"

a. History

Ask	Rationale
Age in hours	To identify onset of illness and etiology
Feeding	Excusive breastfeeding has multiple benefits. Inadequate or insufficient feeding predispose to infection, hypoglycemia and poor weight gain. Top feeds, pre-lacteals also predispose to infection. Lactational failure in previous pregnancy predisposes to recurrence

Contd...

Contd...

Maternal illness	Maternal diabetes predisposes infant to LGA, hypoglycemia, RDS, birth trauma, polycythemia and congenital anomalies. Maternal PIH or eclampsia predisposes to asphyxia, IUGR and thrombocytopenia. Chronic illness in mother may lead to LBW or IUGR baby. Maternal bleeding may cause anemia, shock or respiratory distress in infant
Maternal fever, chorioamnionitis, PROM >12 hours, PPROM, multiple PV examinations	Are risk factors for sepsis?
Difficult labor, prolonged labor, instrumental delivery, fetal distress, need for resuscitation at birth	Are risk factors for asphyxia?
Preterm labor, no antenatal steroids to mother	Predispose to respiratory distress syndrome
Amniotic fluid volume	Polyhydramnios should alert to congenital diaphragmatic hernia, tracheoesophageal fistula, obstructive uropathy. Oligohydramnios is associated with IUGR, post-datism, membrane rupture, pulmonary hypoplasia, and renal agenesis
Family history	Unexplained neonatal deaths, sibling deaths predispose to metabolic, genetic, immunologic or intrauterine infections. Previous preterm labor predisposes to prematurity
Vitamin K to baby	Protects from early, classical and late hemorrhagic disease of newborn
Urine–stool pattern	Not passed urine or stool over 48 hours of birth is worrisome. Indirect parameter to assess breastfeeding adequacy. High-colored urine staining the diapers and pale stools may suggest cholestasis
Infant behavior	Well baby sleeps well, is alert and active when awake. Decreased feed, persistent sleepiness is worrisome
Vaccination	Protection from illness

Abbreviations: LGA, large for gestational age; RDS, respiratory distress syndrome; IUGR, intrauterine growth restriction; LBW, low birth weight; PROM, premature rupture of membrane; PPROM, preterm premature rupture of membrane

ASSESS FOR JAUNDICE SEVERITY

Focused Examination

- Vital parameters
- Pallor or plethora and severity
- Jaundice (cephalocaudal progression). Are palms and soles affected?

- Splenomegaly
- Blood collections (e.g. cephalhematoma, sub-galeal bleed, echymosis)
- Bilirubin-induced neurologic dysfunction (BIND) scoring

Variable/Score	0	1	2	3
Mental status	Normal	Sleepy, difficult to wake	Very sleepy or irritable	Semi-coma, apnea, seizures
Muscle tone	Normal	Mild hypotonia	Moderate hypotonia, arching on stimulus	Persistent arching and opisthotonus
Cry	Normal	High pitched	Shrill	Inconsable or weak or absent
Gaze	Normal			Sun-set or absent superior gaze

Total Score:

Focused Investigations

- Blood group
- Reticulocyte count
- Direct Coombs' test
- Peripheral smear
- Glucose-6-phosphate dehydrogenase (G6PD) deficiency
- Sepsis screen only when clinically indicated

RESPIRATORY DISTRESS

Physical Assessment

Look	Rationale
Sensorium	Increased work of breathing in alert baby is respiratory distress and with worsening sensorium is respiratory failure. Abnormal sensorium is persistent irritability, lethargy or drowsiness
Color	Stable baby has pink color. Altered color pale (anemia, shock), plethora (polycythemia), dusky (cold stress, hypothermia, CHD, shock), cyanosis (cold stress, CHD, respiratory failure) give clue to underlying problem
Tone/posture	A stable baby is active with good tone and responds to pain. Abnormal tone is reflected by posture (frog legged posture, extended posture) and suggests neurologic compromise
Response to touch	Nonresponsive to touch (e.g. Dstix, IV insertion) is ominous and suggests brain dysfunction
Cry	A stable baby has lusty cry. Weak, absent or shrill cry is ominous and suggests neuromuscular weakness

Contd...

Contd...

Vital parameters (Temperature, HR, RR, BP, SpO$_2$)	To define the baseline status, to monitor the trend, to anticipate problems and identify complications
Work of breathing (Downes score or Silverman-Anderson score)	To objectively define respiratory distress, monitor the trend and anticipate deterioration
Perfusion (HR, color, core-axillary temperature, CRT, urine output, BP)	To identify early shock. Monitor the trends. More the parameters abnormal, more is the possibility of shock. Fall in BP (hypotension) is late sign of shock and is a ominous sign
Gestation	Preterms (<34 weeks) are at risk for RDS and rarely develop MAS. Post-terms are at risk for MAS. Late preterm (34–37 weeks) are vulnerable population
Weight	SGA and LGA are at risk for difficult delivery and MSAF
Danger signs (grunt, cyanosis, worsening sensorium, apnea)	To identify life-threatening events and consider urgent transfer/interventions

Abbreviations: CHD, congenital heart disease; IV, intravenous; HR, heart rate; RR, respiratory rate; BP, blood pressure; SpO$_2$, oxygen saturation; CRT, capillary refill time; RDS, respiratory distress syndrome; MAS, meconium aspiration syndrome; SGA, small for gestational age; LGA, large for gestational age; MSAF, meconium stained amniotic fluid.

Respiratory Distress Evaluation: Inspection

SGA	MAS, asphyxia, polycythemia
LGA	Birth trauma, asphyxia, polycythemia, RDS, CHD, Hypoglycemia
Potter facies	Hypoplastic lungs
Barrel chest	MAS
Large caput, bruises	Difficult labor, prolonged labor predisposes to asphyxia
Frothing at mouth	TEF
Meconium staining	MAS
Pallor	Anemia, Shock
Plethora	Polycythemia
Cyanosis	CHD, severe lung disease, shunt, abnormal hemoglobin, air leak
Murmur, hepatomegaly, cardiomegaly, abnormal pulses, differential cyanosis	CHD, shunt

Contd...

Contd...

Fever, hypothermia, cold stress, umbilical sepsis, foul smell, pustules, discharge, petechiae, bleeding tendency, sclerema	Sepsis, pneumonia
Twins	Twin to twin transfusion
Inability to pass orogastric tube	TEF
Isolated cleft palate	Aspiration syndrome
Scaphoid abdomen, distal heart sounds, shift of heart sounds, ipsilateral decreased air entry	Congenital Diaphragmatic Hernia
Temperature instability, core periphery temperature difference >3°C	Pneumonia
Absent femoral pulses	Coarctation of aorta
Cardiomegaly	CHD, cardiomyopathy
Palpation: Tracheal deviation, displaced apical beat, and thrill	
Auscultation: Assess air entry, breath sounds, adventitious sounds	

Abbreviations: SGA, small for gestational age; LGA, large for gestational age; RDS, respiratory distress syndrome; CHD, congenital heart disease; MAS, meconium aspiration syndrome; TEF, tracheoesophageal fistula.

SHOCK

Assessment for Shock

Look	*Rationale*
Sensorium	Abnormal sensorium is persistent irritability, lethargy or drowsiness. Worsening sensorium is an ominous sign
Color	Stable baby has color pink. Altered color (pale- (anemia, shock), plethora (polycythemia), dusky (cold stress, hypothermia, CHD, shock), cyanosis (cold stress, CHD, respiratory failure) gives clue to underlying problem
Tone/posture	A stable baby is active with good tone and responds to pain. Abnormal tone is reflected by posture (frog legged posture, extended posture) and suggests neurologic compromise
Vital parameters (Temperature, HR, RR, BP, SpO$_2$)	To define the baseline status, to monitor the trend, to anticipate problems and identify complications

Contd...

Contd...

Work of breathing (e.g. Downe's score or Silverman Anderson score)	To objectively define respiratory distress, monitor the trend and anticipate deterioration. Adequate oxygenation and ventilation is needed for adequate circulation
Perfusion (HR, color, core-axillary temperature, CRT, urine output, BP)	To identify early shock. Monitor the trends. More the parameters abnormal, more is the possibility of shock. Fall in BP (hypotension) is late sign of shock and is an ominous sign
Gestation	Blood pressure norms vary with postanatal age and gestational age. Very preterm (<28 weeks) are more at risk for hypotension due to immaturity
Danger signs (grunt, cyanosis, worsening sensorium, apnea, hypotension, weak pulses)	To identify life threatening events and consider urgent transfer/interventions
Clinical clues to etiology of shock	
Murmur, hepatomegaly, cardiomegaly, abnormal pulses, differential cyanosis	Cardiogenic shock
Fever, hypothermia, cold stress, umbilical sepsis, foul smell, pustules, discharge, petechiae, bleeding tendency, sclerema	Septic shock
Loss of blood, fluids - internal or external	Hypovolemic shock
Post resuscitation deterioration, sudden deterioration	Obstructive shock
Encephalopathy, weak cry, depressed reflexes, shallow breathing, vasomotor instability	Neurogenic shock

Abbreviations: CHD, congenital heart disease; HR, heart rate; RR, respiratory rate; BP, blood pressure; SpO_2, oxygen saturation; CRT, capillary refill time.

HYPOGLYCEMIA

Assessment of Hypoglycemic Neonate

Note	*Rationale*
Appearance	Small for gestational age (weight <10th percentile) have low glycogen, inadequate hormone and enzyme response, hyperinsulinemia or feeding intolerance. Macrosomia or weight >4.5 kg may be seen in infant of diabetic mothers have hyperinsulinemia

Contd...

Activity	Irritability, jitteriness, seizures, drowsiness or lethargy suggests symptomatic infant
Plethora	Polycythemia (venous Hct >65%) predisposes to hypoglycemia
Cold stress, hypothermia	Thermal instability increases use of glucose, stimulation of catecholamines
Sepsis features (e.g. thermal instability, poor perfusion, core-axillary mismatch, altered sensorium, respiratory distress, etc)	Leads to Inadequate responses of hormone and enzyme, feeding intolerance
Hepatomegaly, microcephaly, anterior midline defects, hemi hypertrophy, macroglossia	Suggest possibility of inborn error of metabolism (IEM)—defects of enzymes gluconeogenesis, glycogenolysis or fatty acid oxidation
Circulatory or respiratory insufficiency	Shift energy metabolism from aerobic to anaerobic pathways: hypoxemia, hypotension, hypoventilation, septic shock

SEIZURES

Assess for Seizures

Day 1 neonate with seizures

a. History

- Note the time of onset (age in hours), type of seizure, associated eye movements, level of consciousness, status, between the episodes
- **Risk factors for asphyxia:** Difficult labor, assisted delivery or precipitate labor, need for resuscitation at birth, fetal distress, and meconium stained liqor
- **Risk factors for sepsis:** Fever, foul smelling liqor, premature rupture of membranes (PROM) >18 hours, uterine tenderness, and maternal antibiotics
- **Family history:** Consanguinity, any affection of sibling or family member with seizures or mental retardation
- **Intrauterine infection:** Maternal fever, rash with lymphadenopathy, previous abortions, maternal intake of alcohol, cocaine, heroin or methadone
- **Feeding:** Frequency, adequacy of breast milk feeding, use of nonhuman milk, worsening noted following feeds.

Bleeding from any site.

b. Examination

- Vitals: Heart rate (HR), respiratory rate (RR), blood pressure (BP), oxygen saturation (SpO$_2$)
- Gestation
- Weight: Small for gestational age (SGA), appropriate for gestational age (AGA) or large for gestational age (LGA)

- Note the type of seizure, involvement of eyes-mouth-limbs, effect on vitals
- Sensorium and cry
- Look for dysmorphic facies, obvious congenital anomalies
- Look for caput, forceps marks, skull fracture, subgaleal bleeds, bulging fontanel, injection site mark on scalp
- Look for neurocutaneous markers like hypopigmented patches
- Significant pallor, plethora, icterus, rash, and bleeding tendency
- Hepatosplenomegaly
- Eye examination for chorioretinitis
- Record any unusual body or urine odor
- Bruit over the anterior fontanel.

c. Stabilization

- Ensure patent airway—sniffing position, suction if necessary
- Attach a multichannel monitor
- Start oxygen by hood at 10 L/min
- Secure intravenous access, do a blood glucose and send for baseline labs (blood sugar, serum ionic calcium, hematocrit (Hct), serum electrolytes, blood culture and sepsis screen as indicated)
- If the bedside sugar is >45 mg%, administer IV phenobarbitone, 20 mg/kg slowly over 30 minutes
- Watch for respiratory depression or recurrence of seizures
- Keep resuscitation apparatus ready
- Consider bedside skull ultrasound
- Consider electroencephalography (EEG) study at earliest
- Assess support and maintain airway, breathing, and circulation
- Counsel parents.

ABNORMAL MOVEMENTS (NOT SEIZURES)

Stabilize the Neonate

- Check temperature, place under radiant warmer if temperature <36.5°C
- Stabilize airway – sniffing position, suction if necessary
- Assess and support breathing (respiratory rate, and work of breathing)
- Circulation - heart rate, rhythm, pulse volume, BP, capillary refill
- Check SpO_2
- Check blood glucose
- Determine if problem is life threatening or non-life threatening
- If life threatening call for help, start resuscitation as per neonatal resuscitation program (NRP).

Evaluate for:

- Gestation
- Vitals: heart rate, breathing and blood pressure
- Observe eye movement
- Observe buccal/oral movements
- Can you stimulate or stop the movement (jitteriness)

- Relation with sleep (benign neonatal sleep myoclonus)
- Association with feeds (gastroesophageal reflux – Sandifer syndrome)
- Neurologic status: Sensorium, tone, posture, reflexes.

A seizure is commonly associated with tachycardia, changes in blood pressure, temperature instability, eye deviation, abnormal limb movement, mouth deviation or abnormal eye opening or closing.

Identify the Problem

- Jitteriness: No eye involvement, can be provoked and stopped, no alteration in vital parameters, disappears in sleep, neurologically normal.
- Benign sleep myoclonus: Always in sleep, neurologically normal, no alteration in vital parameters.
- Hyperekplexia: Can be provoked by tactile and auditory stimuli, may be aborted by flexion of limbs and neck of the newborn, characterized by generalized stiffness while awake, exaggerated startle and nocturnal myoclonus.
- Jaw myoclonus: Trembling of chin.
- Benign paroxysmal torticollis of infancy: Retrocollis, torticollis with abnormal ocular movements with normal sensorium between attacks.
- Classify as seizure: Multifocal clonic movements, tonic posturing, lip smacking, cycling, pedaling, vacant stare associated with autonomic disturbances.

Intervene

- Jitteriness: Look for hypothermia, hypoglycemia, hypoxic-ischemic encephalopathy, hypocalcemia, drug withdrawal, and treat accordingly. Reassure parents.
- Benign paroxysmal torticollis of infancy—get EEG (remits by 5 years of age)
- Hyperekplexia: Vigevano maneuver—flexing baby at neck and hips is used to abort the episode -get EEG (use of clonazepam to prevent hypoxic brain injury)
- Paroxysmal tonic upgaze of childhood: Neuroimaging, EEG (low dose levodopa, and carbidopa)
- Jaw myoclonus: Reassure parents
- Seizures: Check glucose, calcium. Anticonvulsants as indicated.

ASSESSING HYDRATION

- **Weight:** Note the trend in weight or compare the weight with previous recording. Loss of weight 5–10% is seen with some dehydration and >10% with severe dehydration.
- **Sensorium:** Restlesness or irritability is seen with some dehydration. Abnormal sleepiness or lethargy is seen with severe dehydration.
- **Anterior fontanel:** The fontanel appears sunken with dehydration.
- **Mucous membrane:** Note the tongue. It appears dry with dehydration and parched with severe dehydration.
- **Eyes:** Sunken eyes are seen with dehydration.

- **Skin turgor:** Pinch the skin over the abdomen between the thumb and index finger and release. Normal skin retracts immediately. With some dehydration, the skin retracts by 2 seconds and with severe dehydration retracts more than 2 seconds.
- **Breathing:** Tachypnea without chest indrawing suggests some dehydration. Shallow or gasping respiration suggests severe dehydration.
- **Pulse:** Low volume with some dehydration. Thready with severe dehydration.
- **Capillary refill:** Slightly delayed with some dehydration and markedly delayed with severe dehydration.
- **Feeding:** Infant with some dehydration sucks vigorously for feed. No or poor suck is seen with severe dehydration.
- **Urine flow:** Decreased with some dehydration and absent with severe dehydration.

Signs of Circulatory Collapse

Note for lethargy, shallow breathing, weak rapid pulse, pale mottled skin, cool or blue extremities, low blood pressure, delayed capillary refill, and sunken anterior fontanel.

Identify the Problem: Classify the dehydration

- **No dehydration (<3% weight loss):** Normal activity, wet mucosa, eyes not sunken, anterior fontanel at level, normal heart rate, respiratory rate, warm extremities, skin turgor goes back immediately, normal urine output.
- **Some dehydration (3–9% weight loss):** Irritable or restless, able to drink. Dry mucosa, tachycardia, good pulses, cool extremities, skin turgor <2 seconds recoil, and reduced urine output.
- **Severe dehydration (>10% weight loss):** Apneic, apathetic, severely malnourished, cold mottled, cyanotic, skin turgor prolonged, dry mucosa, deeply sunken eyes, and markedly reduced urine output.

Identify Cause for Dehydration

- **Faulty feeding:** Check position, attachment, and milk output
- **Diarrhea:** Top fed/breast fed infant. Is it cholera? (watery stools, increased frequency)
- **Polyuria:** (Renal tubular disorder, neonatal diabetes)
- **Vomiting:** Bilious/nonbilious.

Intervene: Treatment of Dehydration

- **No/minimal dehydration:** Breastfeeding, ORS
- **Some dehydration:** 10% correction, replacement of ongoing losses + maintenance fluids. Evaluation of etiology
- **Severe dehydration:** 15% correction, replacement of ongoing losses + maintenance fluid. Evaluation of etiology
- **Investigations:** Electrolytes, glucose, blood gas, urea, creatinine.

Treatment of Etiology

- **Faulty feeding:** Teach position and attachment, expressed breast milk. Avoid bottle feeds. Monitor weight

- **Diarrhea:** Education on hygiene, evaluation of cause, nutrition, breast feeding, and zinc
- **Polyuria:** Evaluation of tubular disorders
- **Vomiting:** Evaluation of medical/surgical disorders [intestinal obstruction or congenital hypertrophic pyloric stenosis (CHPS)].

Comment

- Clinical assessment of dehydration can be difficult in newborn period and rarely predicts the exact degree of dehydration accurately
- Combinations of signs provide more information than any individual signs in assessing the degree of dehydration.

EXCESSIVE CRYING
Identify "Danger Signs"

- Poor weight gain
- Poor or decreased feeding, change in behavior, vomiting, alternating drowsiness, decreased urination or bloody stools
- Decreased responsiveness
- Documented fever
- Unconsolable cry for two or more hours
- Crying as a result of post injury or fall
- Abnormal movements
- Bruises or swelling over the body
- Turns blue, mottled, or very pale
- History: Vague, evolving, contradictory or changing (not consistent with clinical findings) delay in seeking care or inappropriate parental behavior.

History

- Onset, duration, diurnal variation
- Status in-between episodes: Active, alert, and drowsy
- Sleep pattern
- Feeding: Breast milk, adequacy, and frequency
- Any illness in family members
- Perinatal problems: Fetal distress, need for resuscitation, NICU stay, and medications
- Crying on handling vs crying when left alone
- Suck-rest-suck cycle
- Vaccination in recent past
- Animal milk: Dilution, and mode of feeding
- Stool pattern, frequency, and odor
- Flatulence, vomiting, diarrhea, feeding problems, and past similar episode.

Examination

- Temperature: Hypo- or hyperthermia
- Respiration: Rate, chest indrawing, alae nasi, color
- SpO_2
- Audible sound: Grunt, stridor, and rales
- Weight gain pattern

- Anterior fontanel: Bulging, sunken
- Stuffed nose, discharge
- Ear: Discharge, redness, and tenderness
- Eyes: Foreign body, discharge, swelling
- Mouth: Oral thrush
- Hernial orifice: Any bulge, tenderness
- Wet: Soiled diapers, color of urine and stool
- Fingers/toes: Hair tourniquet, boil
- Skin: Eczema, scabies
- Abnormal posturing
- Abnormal movements of eyes-limb
- Swelling or break in continuity over bones
- Unexplained lesions, fractures, and bruises
- Palpable lump in abdomen
- Swollen scrotum
- Unexplained hepatomegaly
- Perfusion: Skin color, skin temperature, capillary refill, pulse volume, urine output
- Pallor, plethora, rash, icterus, bleeding from any site
- Fundus: Retinal hemorrhage
- Parental response, reaction.

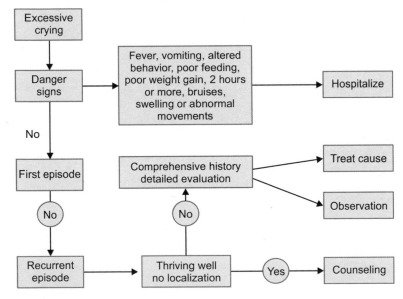

Flowchart 3.1: Action plan for newborn with excessive crying

VOMITING

Exclude Emergency First

- Assess for airway, breathing, circulation and dextrose
- Assess hydration
- Critical diagnosis in mind while taking focused history and doing examination

a. Surgical causes of vomiting (malrotation)
b. Congenital adrenal hyperplasia (CAH)
c. Central nervous system (CNS) causes—intracranial hemorrhage, meningitis.

History

- Onset, duration, frequency
- Color: Bilious, bloody merits hospitalization
- Feeding pattern: Breast milk (adequacy and frequency), nonhuman milk, dilution of feeds, and mode of feeding
- Status between vomiting episodes
- Stool consistency, frequency, and color
- Relation with feed or without feed
- Abdominal fullness or change in contour
- Relation with passage of urine or stool
- Unexplained sibling or family member deaths
- Prenatal: Polyhydramnios, anomaly scans, fetal distress, and intrauterine growth restriction (IUGR)

Examination

- Sensorium: Alert, active, drowsy, lethargy
- Weight pattern
- Fever suggests infection
- HR: Tachycardia, bradycardia
- RR: Tachypnea, shallow breathing, work of breathing
- BP: Hypo- or hypertension
- Hydration: Anterior fontanel, eyes, mucous membranes, feed, skin turgor, and urine frequency
- P/A: Consistency, palpable lump, loop in abdomen, organomegaly, and bowel sounds
- CNS: AF, sensorium, abnormal movements, and abnormal cry
- Odor to urine or body.

PREVIOUS SIBLING UNEXPECTED DEATH

History

1. Sequence of events before the death of the newborn
   a. Vomitings, altered sensorium, seizures, fast breathing, rapid deterioration, normal at birth and first 48 hours: EIM
   b. Decreased activity, dullness, mottled, pallor, fast breathing, cold peripheries, normal at birth and first few days: Duct dependent CHD
   c. Well in the first one or two weeks, vomitings, poor feedings, mottled, hyperpigmentation of genitals and axilla, suggestion of electrolyte imbalance: CAH
   d. Sudden death : No preceding history or illness : Prolonged QTc
   e. Early morning death usually after four weeks : Fatty acid oxidation defects or glycogen storage disorders.

Examination

a. Observation for first few days
b. Genitals: hyperpigmentation, ambiguity
c. Penis size
d. Soft hepatomegaly and mild tachypnea
e. Vomitings and not regurgitations
f. Femoral pulses
g. Baseline tests (e.g. random blood sugar, electrolytes, electrocardiogram, newborn screening (acyl carnitine profile)

COUGH IN A NEONATE

1. Stabilize and assess

- Check temperature, place under radiant warmer if temperature < 36.5°C
- Stabilize airway—sniffing position, suction airway if necessary
- Breathing (respiratory rate, work of breathing)
- Circulation—heart rate, rhythm, pulse volume, BP, capillary refill, core axillary temperature
- Check SpO_2
- Check blood glucose
- Determine if problem is life threatening or non-life threatening
- If life threatening call for help, start resuscitation as per NRP.

2. Focused history

- Gestation, age, birth weight, mode of delivery
- Onset and duration of cough (e.g. acute onset with aspiration, insidious with diphtheria)
- Relationship to feeding (aspiration/reflux/tracheoesophageal fistula)
- Other triggers
- Associated symptoms (fever, poor feeding, sweating, cyanosis, rash)
- Nature of cough (paroxysms/whoop)
- Post-tussive vomiting
- Family history (recent febrile/respiratory illness, congenital anomalies)
- Immunization (mother vaccinated against diphtheria)
- Medications (angiotensin-converting enzyme inhibitors).

3. Focused clinical examination

- Chest shape, symmetry and movement
- Count respiratory rate for 1 minute
- Listen and auscultate (air entry, murmur, adventitious sounds—stridor/grunt/wheeze/crackles)
- Precordial pulsation.

4. Summarize assessment and plan

- Gestation, weight, AGA, SGA or LGA
- General condition and physical findings
- Differential diagnoses
- Investigation and treatment plan.

5. Counsel parents

- Encourage parents to ask questions and voice concerns
- Summarize using lay person's terms and local language (get translator if needed)
- Be patient, polite, and empathetic.

CASE STUDIES: JAUNDICE

Case 1

A 34-week neonate born to mother with Rh negative pregnancy with birth weight of 2 kg. The cord blood TSB was 5.8 mg/dL and hematocrit was 25. Mother blood group was O negative while baby was B positive.

Questions

1. What is the next step?
2. How do you calculate required blood volume required for double volume exchange transfusion (DVET)?
3. Write 3 common complications associated with DVET.

Answers

1. Initial examination should focus at assessing hemodynamic status and then.
   a. Plan for partial exchange transfusion with O negative PRBC at 50 mL/kg.
   b. Also plan for DVET as TSB is 5.8 mg/dL, after stabilizing the neonate.
2. First calculate the blood volume of the baby based on Rawling's chart and double it

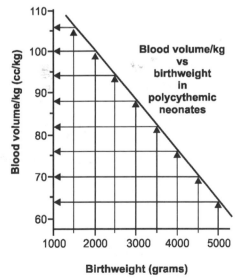

Fig. 1: Nomogram designed for clinical use correlating blood volume (BV)/kg with birth weight in polycythemic neonates

In this case, the blood volume required is 2 × 100 = 200 mL
PRBC required (70%): 140 mL of O negative
FFP required (30%): 60 mL of AB group;

Note: In case of unavailability of above charts, one can calculate by assuming blood volume as 80 mL/kg.

3. The common complications after DVET are metabolic disturbance like hypocalcemia, hypoglycemia/hyperglycemia, hyperkalemia and acidosis. Apart from these baby can also have following:
   - Arrhythmias
   - Respiratory and hemodynamic instability
   - Air embolism
   - Blood transfusion associated infections
   - Necrotising enterocolitis
   - Graft vs host disease

Case 2

A 2.8 kg, baby boy is born to a primigravida mother following uneventful delivery. The infant is noticed to be deep jaundice at 70 hours of age and is irritable. The maternal blood group is A Rh –ve, infant is O Rh +ve with serum bilirubin (total) of 21 mg%. You decide to perform exchange transfusion (ET).

Questions

1. What is your preferred blood for ET in this boy?
2. Name four clinical features that would indicate need for ET irrespective of bilirubin value.
3. Name two hazards of using old blood for ET.
4. What is the percentage of blood replaced by single and double volume ET?
5. Name two contraindications for placement of umbilical catheter.
6. What is cold heart syndrome?
7. How much volume of blood should be removed/infused per aliquot?
8. How much rebound bilirubin rise is likely to occur by 30 minutes post procedure>
9. What is the choice of antibiotic to be given for ET?
10. Name four risk factors which predispose to early neurotoxicity with low bilirubin.
11. Name two hematological complications of ET.
12. Name a maneuver that you perform every 5–10 cycles during ET to ensure consistent hematocrit.
13. Name a cardiovascular drug, which is known to displace bilirubin.

Answers

1. Type O negative packed red blood cells (RBCs) with low anti-A and anti-B titers and reconstituted in AB plasma, cross matched against infant and mothers blood.
2. Hypertonia, arching, retrocollis, opisthotonos, fever, high pitched cry—acute bilirubin encephalopathy
3. Hyperkalemia, acidosis, thrombocytopenia
4. 63% and 86%

5. Omphalitis, malformation of cord (gastroschisis, omphalocele), patent urachus, NEC, age >1–2 weeks
6. Cold heart syndrome is thought to be related to cold blood and high potassium(Kþ) values. It may lead to arrhythmia and cardiac arrest.
7. 5 cc/kg ((not to exceed 10% of the total blood volume)
8. Approximately 60% of the pre-exchange levels.
9. No antibiotic is needed for the procedure.
10. Prematurity, hemolytic disease, G6PD deficiency, asphyxia, sepsis, acidosis, and hypoalbuminemia (<3 g/dL)
11. Anemia, thrombocytopenia, hemorrhage
12. Gentle shaking or kneading) of the donor blood bag
13. Ibuprufen.

Case 3

A 2.1 kg baby boy is born to a primigravida mother following uneventful delivery at 34 weeks gestation. At 31 hours they are discharged. There were no other complaints. The infant is noticed to have deep jaundice at 70 hours of age and is irritable. The maternal blood group is A Rh –ve, infant is O Rh +ve with serum bilirubin of 21 mg% and weight of 2 kg. You decide to perform exchange transfusion (ET).

Questions
1. Name five errors that were made in the care of this newborn.
2. Name five risk factors that contributed to hyperbilirubinemia in this case.

Answers
1. No assessment of lactation adequacy, ignoring the risk factors for jaundice (e.g. primi, nearterm, LBW, lactational insufficiency, maternal blood group), not knowing the maternal blood group, relying on visual assessment for jaundice at discharge, not screening by Tc or TSB at discharge, not informing when to follow up, not informing the danger signs for jaundice, early discharge without ensuring maternal confidence in caring, thorough assessment of newborn (history/exam) was missed.
2. Gestational age 34 weeks, Primi, Rh incompatibility setting, Exclusive breastfeeding, inadequacy of feeding, male baby.

Case 4

A 2.1 kg baby boy is born to a primigravida mother following uneventful delivery at 34 weeks gestation. At 31 hours they are discharged. There were no complaints. You find some jaundice upto trunk. Mother is O Rh +ve. You identify this as a high-risk baby for hyperbilirubinemia.

Questions
1. What is the risk period to develop significant jaundice?
2. When should you schedule a follow up for this infant?

3. What best action you should take at time of birth for objective assessment of jaundice?
4. Name four parameters you assess on follow up of this infant.

Answers

1. First 96 hours of life
2. Being discharged within 48 hours of life, follow up should be scheduled within 48–72 hours and between 72 and 180 hours with clear written and verbal instructions.
3. TcB or TSB and plotting on hour specific bilirubin chart to define the severity of jaundice.
4. Assess weight, percent change in weight from birth weight, adequacy of intake, voiding and stooling, presence/absence of jaundice.

Case 5

A 2.1 kg baby boy is born to a primigravida, O Rh +ve following an uneventful delivery at 36 weeks of gestation. At 72 hours he is active, TcB is 14 mg%. His blood group is A Rh –ve. Total serum bilirubin is 18 mg%. You decide to initiate phototherapy (PT).

Questions

1. What is the etiology of jaundice?
2. Name three key aspects that increase efficiency of phototherapy.
3. Name three mechanisms by which phototherapy works.
4. Which phototherapy can be brought closest to the infant?
5. Name three drawbacks of Tc bilirubin.
6. What is the irradiance level for standard phototherapy?
7. Which PT lamps have the longest life span?
8. Name two conditions where a check for TSB is done 24 hours of stopping PT for rebound jaundice.
9. Name the components of BIND score.
10. What is failure of PT?

Answers

1. ABO incompatibility.
2. Irradiance, wavelength of light, body surface area.
3. Photo-oxidation, structural isomerization, configurational isomerization.
4. Fibreoptic PT.
5. Not for <34 week infants, not <24 hours, screening tool not a therapeutic tool, not reliable in dark and PT exposed infants, and need calibration.
6. 8–12 uW/cm^2/nm.
7. Blue LED, at least 3000 hours.
8. <37 weeks, +ve DCT, bruising.
9. Sleep state, mental, tone and cry.
10. Inability to observe a decline in bilirubin of 1–2 mg/dL after 4–6 hours and/or to keep the bilirubin below the exchange transfusion level.

Case 6

A 38-week neonate born to primigravida mother with a birth weight of 3 kg by normal vaginal delivery. He was found to have jaundice at 24 hours of life and TSB was 14 mg/dL. The baby was shifted to neonatal intensive care unit (NICU) and started on phototherapy. After 6 hours, TSB was found to be 22 mg/dL. Baby's blood group was A positive, reticulocyte count was 8%, direct Coombs test (DCT) was positive and packed cell volume (PCV) was 38%.

1. What is the next step?
2. If you want to go for DVET, which blood group's blood you will choose?
3. The baby developed abnormal movements and lethargy after exchange transfusion.

What are the common causes for this condition?

Answers

1. The management includes:
   - Continue intensive phototherapy and check the irradiance
   - Arrange blood for DVET
   - Counsel and take consent from the parents regarding the procedure
2. The blood should be a mixture of 'O' positive packed red blood cells (PRBC) and AB plasma in 70:30 ratio and cross-matched with mother and baby's blood sample
3. Most common causes for the above condition are hypoglycemia and hypocalcemia.

CASE STUDIES: RESPIRATORY DISTRESS

Case 1

30 week, 1.2 kg infant born to primigravida mother with no prenatal risk factors. The baby developed tachypnea and grunting immediately after birth. Mother received 1 dose of dexamethasone 8 hours prior to delivery. Identify the measures that you would take to stabilize this newborn from the findings noted in the newborn?

Finding	Plan
a. SA score 3	1. Consider surfactant
b. No change in FiO_2 over 6 hours	2. CPAP failure likely
c. FiO_2 0.4	3. Hiflow oxygen
d. Recurrent apnea	4. Early CPAP
e. White out X-ray chest	5. Initiate ventilation
	6. Repeat surfactant
	7. Prophylactic CPAP

Answers: a–4, b–6, c–1, d–5, e–2

Case 2

A term infant born to a primigravida mother with antenatal polyhydramnios is noted to be apneic at birth. Despite corrective measures with positive pressure ventilation the baby remains blue. You intubate the baby following which there is improvement. You find heart sounds best heard along right sternal border. You decide to transfer the baby to NICU with ongoing ventilation support.

Questions

1. What is the most likely diagnosis?
2. Why did this newborn not respond to bag and mask ventilation?
3. Name two most important underlying conditions which influence the timing of presentation and clinical outcome postnatal.
4. Name two prenatal predictors for poor outcome.

Answers

1. Congenital diaphragmatic hernia.
2. Intestines occupying the thoracic cage become distended with air following bag and mask which further compromises pulmonary function.
3. Pulmonary hypoplasia and pulmonary hypertension.
4. Liver herniation, stomach and spleen in chest on left side, >50% liver in chest on right side, and observed to predicted (O/E) lung area to head circumference ratio (LHR) <25%.

Case 3

You are asked to evaluate a newborn, 1 hour of age, with respiratory distress. You find copious salivation. There is fullness of abdomen. Bilateral noisy sounds are heard in the chest. You shift the newborn to NICU. A chest X-ray is done.

Questions

1. What is the chromosomal association with this condition?
2. What are the other associations of this condition?
3. What decides the risk of complications post surgery in such an infant?
4. What is the risk of recurrence with isolated defect?

Answers

1. Trisomy 21 (double bubble shadow s/o duodenal atresia)
2. VACTERL (vertebral, anorectal, cardiac, tracheoesophageal, renal, and limb defects) or CHARGE (Coloboma, Heart defects, Atresia choanae, Retarded development, Genital hypoplasia, Ear abnormalities)
3. "Long gap" repairs (more than two vertebral bodies or more than 3 cm).
4. <1%.

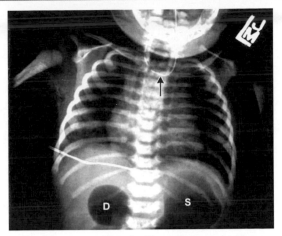

Fig. 2: Chest X-ray

Case 4

This term newborn is noted to have progressive respiratory distress immediately after birth.

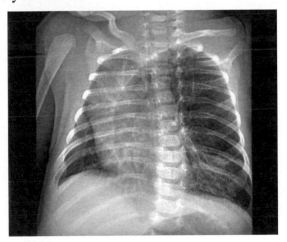

Fig. 3

Questions

1. What is the diagnosis?
2. Name the investigation of choice to confirm this condition?
3. What is the definitive treatment for this condition?
4. The infant becomes blue during anesthesia induction. Why?

Answers

1. Left congenital lobar overinflation (emphysema)
2. CT thorax
3. Lobectomy/surgery

4. These patients may not tolerate positive pressure ventilation which can lead to air trapping, air leak and rarely a cardiac arrest

Case 5

An intubated term newborn with respiratory distress abruptly becomes blue.

Questions

1. Name the four most common causes for this condition.
2. What noninvasive procedure do you perform to confirms clinical diagnosis?
3. Why do you need to take a cross table lateral view X-ray chest?

Answers

1. DOPE-displaced tube, obstructed tube, pneumothroax, and equipment failure
2. Trans-illumination of chest
3. To define anterior air leaks (retrosternal) and define the position of ICD.

Case 6

A post-term newborn with meconium stained liquor has progressive respiratory distress immediately after birth. You notice there is a grunt.

Questions

1. What does grunt signify?
2. Name two most common complications for this condition.
3. Below what gestational age is this condition rarely seen?

Answers

1. Grunting happens when the infant attempts to keep the alveoli open to maintain the functional residual capacity by partially closing the glottis during expiration.
2. Air leak syndromes, PPHN.
3. <34 weeks.

CASE STUDIES: SICK NEWBORN

Case 1

A 30 week 1.3 kg infant presents at 2 hours of age with poor perfusion. Mother had history of PPROM for 16 hours.

1. What is the role of sepsis screen in such an infant on admission?
2. What is the gold standard for blood pressure measurement?
3. Which is the most reliable clinical feature to suggest poor perfusion?
4. What is permissive hypotenion?

Answers

1. No role.
2. Invasive BP.

3. No clinical feature in isolation is reliable to suggest poor perfusion. A combination of signs and more importantly the trend is most informative.
4. A low BP reading in an otherwise well baby with no signs of poor perfusion. It merits monitoring but no intervention.

Case 2

A term neonate delivered by forceps application is brought with seizures at 6 hours of age. On examination he had decreased movements of left upper limb, pinpoint pupils and bradycardia.

Questions

1. What is the HIE staging (Sarnat and Sarnat) of this baby?
2. Name two most common causes for decreased movements of left upper limb.
3. How to differentiate Erbs from Klumpe palsy clinically?

Answers

1. Stage II.
2. Left Erb's palsy, left clavicular fracture.
3. The grasp reflex is preserved in Erbs palsy.

Case 3

Term, 1.8 kg, infant is asymptomatic. There were no risk factors during pregnancy and the delivery was uneventful. You are concerned about hypoglycemia.

Questions

1. What is the upper age limit to screen for hypoglycemia in "at risk" newborns?
2. What is the difference between blood and plasma glucose?
3. Which clinical sign is most specific for hypoglycemia?
4. What is differential hypoglycemia?

Answers

1. 72 hours
2. Glucose concentration measured in whole blood is 10–15% lower than that in plasma.
3. No clinical signs is specific for hypoglycemia. Hypoglycemia is not a clinical diagnosis. It is a biochemical diagnosis.
4. Some infants with glucose being infused through an umbilical artery line may have normal glucose levels in their feet but hypoglycemic levels in the hands and brain.

Case 4

A 46-hours-old male neonate with a birth weight of 1.9 kg was brought to the emergency with lethargy. Baby was born to primigravida mother at 39 weeks of gestation who is a known case of type 1 diabetes mellitus.

Questions

1. What are the possibilities for significant lethargy in this infant?

On examination, head circumference was 33 cm; length: 48 cm and chest circumference was 29 cm; Baby was found to be plethoric and peripheries were cool; Axillary temperature was 36.6°C, heart rate was 164 per min and respiratory rate was 46 per minutes.

2. Calculate the ponderal index and classify the type of IUGR in this baby.

3. What are the important investigations you will do for this baby and specify the reason?

4. What is the advice you give at discharge?

Answers

1. The possible causes of lethargy in this neonate are:
   a. Metabolic disturbances like hypoglycemia and hypocalcemia
   b. Hypothermia
   c. Sepsis
   d. Encephalopathy due to polycythemia
2. Ponderal index and the type of IUGR are:
   a. PI = 1.8
   b. PI <2; HC and length are spared; suggests asymmetric IUGR;
3. The important investigations and the reasons are:
   a. Random blood sugar: To rule out hypoglycemia (IUGR newborns are born with limited in utero stores).
   b. Hematocrit/PCV: To rule out polycythemia (IUGR increase the erythropoietin production in utero).
   c. Septic screen: lethargy and cool peripheries.
4. Advice at discharge should include prevention of hypoglycemia, hypothermia and infections
   a. Emphasis on feeding including supplemental feeding.
   b. Prevention of hypothermia with kangaroo mother care and adequate clothing.
   c. Danger signs and early signs of sepsis to be explained.

4

Case Studies

Case 1

D2, term baby is jittery. He has loud ejection systolic murmur radiating to axilla. X-ray Chest, B sugar is normal. S. calcium is 13 mg/dL. 2D Echo shows bilateral pulmonary branch stenosis with a supravalvular aortic narrowing.

Questions

1. What is the diagnosis?
2. What is the likely natural history of the supravalvular aortic and bilateral pulmonary branch stenosis?

Answers

1. Williams syndrome (7q11.23 deletion)
2. The supravalvular aortic stenosis will worsen and the pulmonary branch stenosis resolve with increasing age.

Case 2

2.4 kg, precipitate delivery, baby is pale with dysmorphism with SpO_2 90% for first 2 days and has a soft systolic murmur. X-ray chest is normal. S. calcium is 7 mg%. 2D Echo on D2 is s/o large subaortic VSD with no identifiable pulmonary valve or main pulmonary artery.

Questions

1. What is the diagnosis?
2. What is the immediate neonatal implications of making the above diagnosis?

Answers

1. DiGeorge/velocardiofacial syndrome (22q11 deletion)
2. Risk of immune deficiency, which has implications for infection, immunization, hypocalcemia and blood transfusion. Cleft palate and soft palate dysfunction are recognized associations of 22q11 deletion.

Case 3

2.8 kg, term, vaginal born, no risk factors for sepsis, has weak cry/ irregular breathing. Needs ventilation for 1 week. X-ray chest, sepsis screen are reported normal. The baby is discharged on day 14 with mild tachypnea. At 6 weeks, he is alert, smiles, has tongue fasciculation, weak cry. Neurological assessment was significant for hypotonia (UL>LL), weakness and depressed tendon reflexes.

Questions

1. What is the probable diagnosis?
2. What is the differential diagnosis?
3. What further tests are needed?
4. What is the prognosis of this condition?

Answers

1. Type 1 spinal muscular atrophy
2. Phrenic nerve injury, diaphragmatic paralysis, spinal muscular atrophy, axonal neuropathy, and myotonic dystrophy
3. Muscle biopsy shows atrophy; electromyelogram shows evidence of denervation and reinnervation; nerve conduction studies, creatine phosphokinase may be normal or only mildly elevated compared with high levels in muscular dystrophies; echocardiogram and genetic testing.
4. This child has signs of type 1 spinal muscular atrophy (Werdnig-Hoffman disease) and will inevitably die, most likely before the age of 18 months

Questions

Match the following conditions with respective mechanism:

No.	Condition	Mechanism
1.	Anencephaly	a. Deformation
2.	Club foot or CTEV	b. Disruption
3.	Amniotic band syndrome	c. Malformation
4.	Osteogenesis Imperfecta	d. Dysplasia
		e. Autosomal recessive
		f. X-linked recessive

Answers: 1-c, 2-a, 3-b, 4-d

Case 4

A day-6-infant on routine evaluation is noticed to have the following over the lower back.

Questions

1. Identify the lesion shown in Figure 1.
2. When is it considered benign?
3. Name four indications for doing an USG spine.

Answer

1. Sacral dimple (Fig. 1)
2. A midline dimple measuring less than 5 mm that is located within 2.5 cm of the anus and not associated with other cutaneous findings is benign and routine spinal ultrasonography is not warranted in these patients.
3. Dimples that are large (>5 mm) or high on the back (>2.5 cm from the anus), overlying hemangioma, cutis aplasia, raised lesions (masses, tail-like appendages, and hairy patches) and the presence of multiple cutaneous lesions.

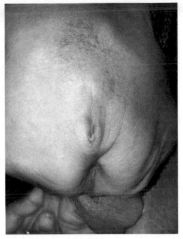

Fig. 1

Case 5

A 1.6 kg, 32-week-infant is clinically stable. In addition to your routine care you wish to initiate kangaroo care (KC).

Questions

1. What are the three basic key components of KC?
2. Kangaroo position is the hallmark of KC. What is kangaroo position?
3. Name four nonthermal benefits to the baby.
4. Which babies are not eligible for KC?

Answers

1. Skin-to-skin contact, exclusive breastfeeding and early discharge
2. Baby in upright position with babies abdomen at level of mother's xiphisternum. Head turned to one side slightly extended with flexed limbs
3. Earlier discharge from nursery, better weight gain, lesser risk of apnea, lesser nosocomial infections, stronger bonding with the mother
4. Sick or unstable babies.

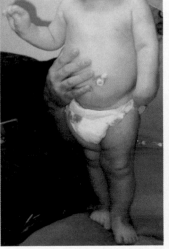
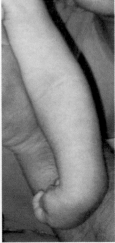

Fig. 2

Observe the clinical photographs (Fig. 2) and answer the following:

Questions

1. What is the diagnosis (Fig. 2)?
2. Name the four components which describe the position of the upper limb
3. Mention any two risk factors for this condition in the newborn.
4. Where is the site of lesion?
5. What are the good prognostic signs?

Answers

1. Duchenne-Erb palsy
2. Shoulder abduction and internal rotation, elbow extension and pronation, wrist and finger flexion (Waiter' tip)
3. Breech, shoulder dystocia, large for gestation, difficult forceps
4. C5, C6, C7
5. Early onset of recovery (within 2–4 weeks of age), unilateral affection, no Klumpe palsy, no involvement of diaphragm.

Pulse Oximetry Predischarge

Questions

1. When pulsoximeter is used as a predischarge screening tool, when is the screening considered positive and what are the interpretations?
2. Name four critical cardiac conditions identified by pulse oximeter?
3. Name four heart defects likely to be missed on screening?

Answers

1. Pulse oximetry screening is done to all newborns at 24 hours after birth. The screening criteria and the interpretations of a positive screen are (three types of positive screens (screening 'failures') are possible that lead to further investigation for the presence of critical congenital heart disease (CCHD)
    - Type 1, universal low saturation: Oxygen saturation < 90% in either limb on a single reading.
    - Type 2, universal borderline saturation: Oxygen saturation of 90–94% in both limbs on three consecutive readings at hourly intervals.
    - Type 3, differential saturation: A difference in the oxygen saturation of 4% or more between the upper and lower limbs on three consecutive readings at hourly intervals.
2. Screening by pulse oximeter identifies the following critical congenital heart disease:
    - Pulmonary atresia
    - Tetralogy of Fallot
    - Transposition of great vessels
    - Truncus arteriosus
    - Tricuspid atresia
    - Total anomalous pulmonary venous return
3. Left to right shunts, coarctation of aorta, interrupted aortic arch, and hypoplastic left heart syndrome.

Management of Child with Clinical Diagnosis of DDH

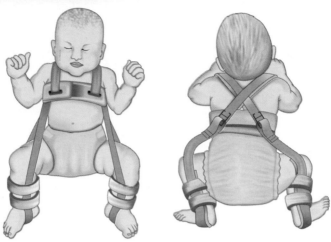

Fig. 3

Questions
1. How do you confirm DDH?
2. Identify the treatment offered to this newborn (Fig. 3).
3. What are the indications for this treatment?
4. What are the contraindications for this treatment?
5. What are the limitations of this procedure?
6. What are the complications of this procedure?

Answers
1. Ultrasound examination: By measuring Graf angle
2. Pavlik harness
3. DDH and fracture femur up to age of 6 months
4. Bilateral DDH
5. The limitations of Pavlik Harness are:
   - If the dislocated hip does not relocate within 3–4 weeks
   - Child over the age of 6 months
   - Large babies
6. The known complications are femoral nerve palsy, avascular necrosis of head of femur and Pavlik disease.

Questions
1. List three disease prevention measures routinely administered to all newborns.
2. List three early disease detection measures which should be routinely administered to all newborns at hospital discharge.
3. Physiologic jaundice is a diagnosis of exclusion (True/false).
4. Name three major physiologic changes that must occur in the newborn shortly after birth in order to transit to extrauterine life.

Answers

1. Vitamin K to prevent late HDN, pulse ox screen to detect critical cyanotic congenital heart defects, hearing screen to detect deafness, vaccinations to prevent severe infections.
2. TcB, SpO_2, metabolic blood screen, OAE screen.
3. True
4. The three events are:
   a. Cord clamping and increased systemic vascular resistance.
   b. Air replaces fluid filled alveoli, increased pulmonary blood flow with drop in pulmonary pressure.
   c. Closure of the shunts (ductus venosus, ductus arteriosus and foramen ovale).

CARDIOLOGY

Case 1

A neonate is brought to the ER at day 28 of life with history of poor feeding and lethargy. On examination the capillary refill time is prolonged but peripheral pulses are feeble. The ECG of the newborn is shown here in Figure 4.

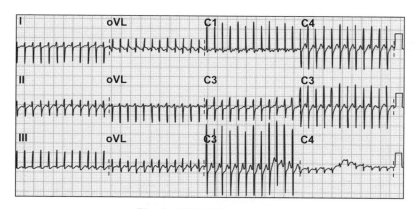

Fig. 4: ECG of the newborn

Questions

1. What is the diagnosis?
2. Name the drug of choice and the dose for medical cardioverison.

Answers

1. Narrow complex supraventricular tachycardia
2. Drug of choice for pharmacologic conversion is adenosine (at the dose of 0.1mg/kg with 2 syringe technique followed by a rapid bolus of 5 mL normal saline).

Case 2

Questions

Write in one word, the name of the receptor/mechanism of action of the following drugs:

1. Milrinone
2. Levosimendan
3. Sildenafil
4. Digoxin
5. Bosentan

Answers

1. Milrinone: Phosphodiesterase 3 inhibitor
2. Levosimendan: Calcium sensitizer
3. Sildenafil: Phosphodiesterase 5 inhibitor
4. Digoxin: Na^+/K^+ ATpase inhibitor
5. Bosentan: Endothelial receptor (A and B) antagonist.

Case 3

Questions

Name the characteristic appearance on X-ray and write the diagnosis.

1. Describe the Figure 5A and the diagnosis.
2. Describe the Figure 5B and the diagnosis.

Answers

1. Egg on string sign: Transposition of great vessels
2. Boot-shaped heart sign: Tetralogy of Fallot

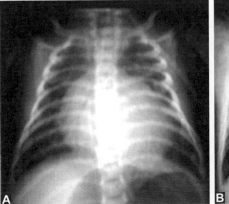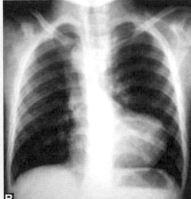

Figs 5A and B

Case 4

A neonate at day 20 of life is rushed to the ER in view of bradycardia. Baby is hemodynamically stable but has tachypnea with a heart rate of 40/min. BP and CRT are maintained. Baby also has fine rashes over the periorbital area.

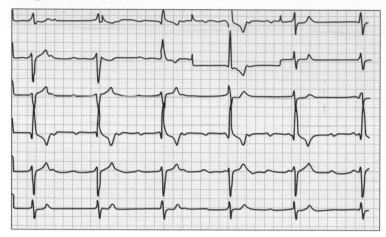

Fig. 6: ECG

Questions
1. What is the ECG diagnosis and probable diagnosis?
2. What is the pathogenesis of the disease?
3. What would be the line of management?

Answers
1. Third degree or congenital complete atrioventricular block (Fig. 6). Probable diagnosis is neonatal Lupus.
2. Autoimmune—passage of maternal anti-Ro and anti-La antibodies to the fetus
3. Stabilize the neonate. Monitor lactates and look for features of CCF. The baby may require very early pacemaker implantation.

Case 5

Questions

1. Name five duct dependent lesions.
2. How do you constitute inj. prostaglandin and write the dose?
3. What are the side effects of prostaglandin for anticipate?

Answers

The duct dependent circulations are:
1. Dependent pulmonary circulation:
    - Tetralogy of Fallot with pulmonary atresia
    - Pulmonary atresia with intact interventricular septum
    - Severe Ebstein's anomaly
    - Critical pulmonary stenosis

Duct dependent systemic circulation
- – Coarctation of aorta, interrupted aortic arch
- – Hypoplastic left heart syndrome
2. Constituting inj. prostaglandin E1 would include
- – Dilute one ampoule (500 µg) in 50 mL D5 or D10 and give as an infusion with dose range of 0.005–0.1 µg/kg/min
3. The side effects of prostaglandin E are: Respiratory depression, hyperthermia, tachycardia, hypotension, seizures, and hypoglycemia.

Case 6

Questions

Name 5 congenital heart defects which can be diagnosed/strongly suspected on pulse oximetry screening.

Answers

1. Transposition of great vessels
2. Tetralogy of Fallot
3. Pulmonary atresia
4. Hypoplastic left heart syndrome
5. Obstructed TAPVC.

Case 7

An abnormal apical four-chamber view of the heart (showing the atrioventricular valves) is seen with many, but not all, forms of congenital heart disease. Which of the following cardiac diagnoses could have a normal four-chamber view?

Questions

1. Hypoplastic left heart syndrome
2. Transposition of the great arteries
3. Tricuspid atresia
4. Ebstein's anomaly of tricuspid valve.

Answer

Transposition of great arteries.

Case 8

Questions

Which of the following forms of congenital heart disease is not a ductal-dependent lesion?

1. Interrupted aortic arch
2. D-transposition of the great arteries
3. Critical aortic stenosis
4. Atrioventricular septal defect.

Answer

4. Atrioventricular septal defect.

ELECTROLYTE DISTURBANCES

Case 1

A 4 days male baby presents with decreased urine output for 2 days. He was born at term with perinatal asphyxia and had seizures on 3rd day of life. His birth weight was 3.5 kg, and current weight is 3.7 kg. His serum electrolytes showed Na^+ of 120 mEq/L, K^+ 5.2 mEq/L, Cl^- 93 mEq/L, and HCO_3^- 17 mEq/L. Blood urea and serum creatinine were 95 mg/dL and 2.2 mg/dL, respectively. RBS was 90 mg/dL, and serum albumin 2.7 g/dL.

Questions

1. What is the etiology of hyponatremia?
2. What are the 3 main clinical groups considered in evaluation of hyponatremia?
3. What is an important clue towards type of hyponatremia?
4. How will you manage this hyponatremia?
5. Is there a role for 3% NaCl?

Answers

1. Hyponatremia is due to AKI stage 3 (decreased GFR that has resulted in impaired water excretion causing water retention and subsequently dilutional hyponatremia)
2. Hyponatremia associated with:
   - Decreased intravascular volume (as with vomiting, diarrhea, sepsis, burns)
   - Euvolemia (SIADH, hypothyroidism, hypocortisolism)
   - Volume overload states (AKI, nephrotic syndrome, cirrhosis, CCF).
3. Weight gain (expected weight loss in first week of life)
4. Fluid restriction, salt restriction, diuretics, and if no improvement, dialysis.
5. No role for 3% NaCl infusion—it may worsen the fluid overload state. The only major indication for 3% NaCl therapy is with symptomatic hyponatremia secondary to SIADH (where the GFR is normal).

Case 2

A 10 days baby girl presents with 3 episodes of generalized tonic-clonic seizures for 1 day. She is born to primigravida mother with birth weight of 2.6 kg and is on exclusive breast feeds. Her current weight is 1.9 kg and she is dehydrated with depressed anterior fontanels. She has normal female genitalia. Serum electrolytes showed Na^+ of 170 mEq/L, K^+ 5.2 mEq/L, Cl^- 136 mEq/L, and HCO_3^- 17 mEq/L. Blood urea and serum creatinine were 395 mg/dL and 5.2 mg/dL, respectively.

Questions

1. What is the etiology of hypernatremia?
2. Name one clinical parameter to rule out diabetes insipidus (DI) and then name the test to confirm DI.

3. What is the first step in management of this baby: Isolyte P/0.45 DNS/NS/ RL solution?
4. What is the most important aspect of management—rate of fluid delivery, type of fluid or monitoring the plasma sodium level?
5. What is the rate of correction of hypernatremia and why this rate?
6. What are the associated metabolic complications of hypernatremic dehydration?
7. How does the kidneys appear on USG, what is the reason for this appearance, what does it mimic, and what happens on follow-up USG?

Answers

1. Factors contributing to hypernatremia are:
   - Decreased breast milk production in first week of primigravida mothers
   - Relatively higher breast milk sodium concentration of 30–50 mEq/L compared to ~10 mEq/L in multigravida mothers.
   - Difficulty latching due to IUGR status and anxious mother.
2. Polyuria (urine volume > 4 mL/kg/hour) in presence of dehydration suggests DI. Low urine osmolality will confirm the diagnosis of DI
3. Isotonic saline administration at 20–30 mL/kg to rapidly expand intravascular volume is the first step irrespective of plasma sodium concentration
4. Monitoring plasma sodium levels every 4–6 hours – most important. Rate and type of fluids to be adjusted based on rate of plasma sodium fall
5. Plasma sodium should fall not more than 8–10 mEq/L/day to prevent cerebral edema
6. Hyperglycemia and hypocalcemia due to end-organ resistance to Insulin and paratharomone respectively
7. Echogenic medullary pyramids due to Tamn-Horsfall protein (concentrated urine due to dehydration) mimics medullary nephrocalcinosis and resolves in 1–4 weeks.

Case 3

1 month baby boy presents with failure to thrive, vomiting, and polyuria. He was born at 37 weeks gestation with birth weight 2.7 kg. He appears dehydrated, has weight of 2.5 kg, and normal male genitalia. Serum electrolytes showed Na^+ of 130 mEq/L, K^+ 2.2 meq/L, Cl^- 90 mEq/L, and HCO_3^- 24 mEq/L. venous blood gas had pH of 7.48, pCO_2 45, and HCO_3 27 mEq/L. Blood urea and serum creatinine were 35 mg/dL and 0.8 mg/dL, respectively.

Questions

1. What are the electrolyte abnormalities?
2. Name three common causes of these abnormalities.
3. What additional information in antenatal history is required?
4. Besides history, name one investigation that will help differentiate the etiologies.
5. What is the diagnosis in this baby?
6. What is the treatment of this condition?
7. What is the long-term outcome?

Answers

1. Hypokalemic, hypochloremic metabolic alkalosis
2. Upper GI obstruction or severe GER, Bartter syndrome, chronic frusemide therapy
3. H/o polyhydramnios (AFI >20 cm) would indicate fetal polyuria that is observed with renal salt or water losing conditions (Bartter syndrome, nephrogenic DI, pseudohypoaldosteronsim)
4. Urinary chloride loses are >20 mEq/L in Bartter syndrome whereas it is <20 mEq/L with nonrenal salt losing states (as with vomiting)
5. Bartter syndrome
6. Treat with oral potassium chloride supplementation, salt supplementation (3% NaCl solution orally), and start ibuprofen or indomethacin after correction of hydration and renal parameters (avoid use in first few weeks of life due to physiologically low GFR).
7. Mental development is normal. Growth restriction, and CKD due to nephrocalcinosis are major complications.

Case 4

1 month baby boy, sibling of a baby with Barter syndrome, presents with failure to thrive, vomiting, and polyuria. He was born at 39 weeks gestation with birth weight 3.7 kg. He appears dehydrated, has weight of 3.5 kg, and normal male genitalia. Pyloric mass is not palpable. Serum electrolytes showed Na^+ of 130 mEq/L, K^+ 2.2 mEq/L, Cl^- 90 mEq/L, and HCO_3^- 24 meq/L. VBG had pH of 7.48, pCO_2 45, and HCO_3 27 mEq/L. Blood urea and serum creatinine were 35 mg/dL and 0.8 mg/dL, respectively. Urinary chloride was 10 mEq/L.

Questions

1. What are the electrolyte abnormalities?
2. Name three common causes of these abnormalities.
3. What additional information in antenatal history is required?
4. What is the investigation that will help differentiate the etiologies?
5. What additional investigation/s required? If the diagnosis is indicated from this special investigation answer Q. 6 and Q. 7?
6. What is the treatment of this condition?
7. What is the long-term outcome?

Answers

1. Hypokalemic, hypochloremic metabolic alkalosis
2. Upper GI obstruction or severe GER (most common), Bartter syndrome, chronic frusemide therapy
3. History of polyhydramnios (AFI >20 cm) would indicate fetal polyuria that is observed with renal salt or water losing conditions (Bartter syndrome, nephrogenic DI, pseudohypoaldosteronsim). AF was adequate at 16 cm
4. Urinary chloride loses are >20 mEq/L in Bartter syndrome whereas it is <20 mEq/L with nonrenal salt losing states (as with vomiting). This neonate had urine chloride loses of 10 mEq/L (low, i.e. kidneys are conserving chloride)

5. Upper GI contrast study (Gastrographin). Severe gastroesophageal reflux grade 4. No evidence of pyloric stenosis
6. Treat with IV Normal saline along with potassium chloride supplementation (IV initially followed by oral for 2–3 weeks depending upon the severity), and specific treatment of GER.
7. Excellent.

Case 5

A 3-week baby boy presents with vomiting for 7 days, breathing difficulty of 3 days, along with low-grade fever and cough of 2 days duration. He was born at term with birth weight of 3.5 kg. Amniotic fluid was adequate. His examination showed malnourished boy with weight of 3 kg, SpO_2 of 98% in room air, "rapid breathing/ respiratory distress", clear chest, no murmur or gallop, and normal male genitalia. Serum electrolytes showed Na^+ of 138 mEq/L, K^+ 2.5 mEq/L, Cl^- 116 mEq/L, and HCO_3^- 15 mEq/L. VBG had pH of 7.23, pCO_2 25, and HCO_3 14 mEq/L. Blood urea and serum creatinine were 35 mg/dL and 0.5 mg/dL, respectively. Complete urine examination had specific gravity of 1010, pH 6.5, no protein, no sugar, and no cells.

Questions

1. What is the cause of breathing difficulty?
2. Describe the metabolic abnormalities.
3. What additional investigations are required? From the findings on the investigations answer subsequent questions?
4. What is the diagnosis?
5. What is the first step in management?
6. What is the long-term complication and prognosis?

Answers

1. Metabolic acidemia and not primary pulmonary or cardiac disease.
2. Hypokalemia with hyperchloremic metabolic acidosis (normal anion gap, anion gap of 7) and adequate respiratory compensation.
3. Spot urine electrolytes to calculate urinary anion gap (urine Na^+ + urine K^+ - urine Cl^-, in this case it is +25)—expected positive that indicates deficiency of ammonium and USG abdomen that may or may not show medullary nephrocalcinosis (absence does not rule out dRTA)
4. Distal renal tubular acidosis (dRTA)
5. To correct hypokalemia with intravenous and oral potassium chloride and only after plasma K^+ is more than 3.2 mEq/L, then to start correcting the metabolic acidemia by using potassium citrate. Rapid correction of metabolic acidemia will drive potassium from ECF to ICF compartment compounding the hypokalemia and precipitate cardiac arrhythmia.
6. Long-term prognosis is excellent if dRTA is diagnosed early and treatment continued lifelong. Growth is normal if diagnosed before two years age.

Case 6

A 3-week baby girl presents with failure to thrive and vomitings for 1 week. There is no diarrhea or seizure. She is born at term with weight of 3.7 kg, and amniotic fluid was adequate. On examination, she is dehydrated with weight of 3.0 kg, and no organomegaly. Serum electrolytes showed Na^+ of 115 mEq/L, K^+ 6.5 mEq/L, Cl^- 76 mEq/L, and HCO_3^- 15 mEq/L. VBG had pH of 7.33, pCO_2 35, and HCO_3^- 16 mEq/L. Blood urea and serum creatinine were 55 mg/dL and 0.5 mg/dL, respectively. Complete urine examination had specific gravity of 1010, pH 5.5, no protein, no sugar, and no cells.

Questions

1. What are the common causes of hyperkalemia?
2. What additional information will assist you in the diagnosis?
3. What confirmatory tests would you order?
4. How will you manage the hyponatremia?
5. What is the phenotype in boys with CAH?

Answers

1. After ruling out hemolyzed blood sample, release of K^+ from cells (hemolysis, rhabdomyolysis), and shift of potassium from ICF to ECF in metabolic acidemia, 2 main causes of hyperkalemia are renal failure and aldosterone deficiency (true) or resistance (pseudohypoaldosteronism)
2. Hyperpigmented skin in both boys and girls and ambiguous genitalia in girls suggest a diagnosis of salt wasting congenital adrenal hyperplasia (true aldosterone deficiency).
3. Blood 17 hydoxy progesterone, serum testosterone (both will be increased with CAH), serum cortisol (decreased with CAH), and serum aldosterone (decreased with CAH).
4. Initial treatment is with dextrose normal saline (DNS) followed by oral salt solution (3% NaCl solution) along with oral fludrocortisone and hydrocortisone.
5. Most boys with salt wasting CAH will have normal male genitalia. If untreated, they will have precocious puberty.

Case 7

A 4 weeks baby girl presents with failure to thrive and vomiting for 1 week. There is no diarrhea or seizure. She is born at term with weight of 3.5 kg. AFI was mildly increased to 24 cm. On examination, she is dehydrated with weight of 3.0 kg, and no organomegaly. Serum electrolytes showed Na^+ of 118 mEq/L, K^+ 6.9 mEq/L, Cl^- 76 mEq/L, and HCO_3^- 15 mEq/L. VBG had pH of 7.33, pCO_2 35, and HCO_3^- 16 mEq/L. Blood urea and serum creatinine were 85 mg/dL and 0.6 mg/dL, respectively. CUE is unremarkable. Spot urine Na^+ is 110, K^+ 10, and Cl^- 116 mEq/L, with FENA of 10%.

Questions

1. What are the metabolic abnormalities in this case?
2. Assuming that the baby girl has normal female genitalia, and renal function normalizes in a day, what is the likely diagnosis?
3. What tests will confirm the diagnosis?
4. Name the types of this condition seen in this newborn.
5. What are the associated features in type 1b of this condition?
6. How will you manage the hyponatremia?
7. Is there a role for oral fludrocortisone in therapy of this condition?
8. What is the prognosis?

Answers

1. Hyponatremia, hyperkalemia, and prerenal AKI (blood urea more elevated than serum creatinine).
2. Salt wasting state due to pseudohypoaldosteronism. True hypoaldosteronism is usually associated with cortisol deficiency as in CAH.
3. Plasma aldosteronse assay (level will be very high).
4. PHA type 1a (renal limited), PHA type 1b (systemic defect in ENaC), type 2 (Gordon syndrome-associated with hypertension and hyperkalemia), and Type 3 (acquired, as in obstructive uropathy, medications, etc.).
5. PHA type 1b patients will have recurrent respiratory infections, and sweating in addition to renal salt wasting.
6. Initial treatment is with dextrose normal saline (DNS) followed by high dose oral salt solution (3% NaCl solution) and potassium exchange resins (in milk +/– retention enema).
7. No role of fludrocortisone
8. Most children with PHA type 1a (renal limited) improve by 1–2 years age due to spontaneous maturation in the mineralocorticoid receptor, increased potassium excretion by potassium channels in distal nephron, and increased salt intake by the child. Children with PHA Type 1b are more difficult to treat and have a relatively poor prognosis.

INFECTIONS IN THE NEWBORN

Case 1

Day 16, term male infant was brought to the emergency with lethargy and poor feeding. In the immediate neonatal period the newborn was treated for suspect sepsis with cefotaxime for 5 days. On preliminary investigations Hb was 12 g/dL, TLC 3400/mm³, neutrophils 79% and platelets 60,000/mm³. Cerebrospinal fluid analysis revealed 249 cells/mm³, 80% polymorphs, sugar 25 mg/dL and a simultaneous blood sugar of 68 mg/dL. The neonate was started with injection piperacillin-tazobactam after the initial evaluation.

Questions

1. Is the choice of antibiotic appropriate: Reason?
2. Is meropenem justifiable in this scenario? Why?
3. CSF culture grows *Klebsiella* sensitive to cephalosporins. Should one step down to inj. cefotaxime or avoid the risk since baby had clinically improved on inj. meropenem?

4. What should be the minimum duration of IV antibiotics? When can one switch from IV to oral antibiotics in this scenario?

Answer

1. No, injection piperacillin-tazobactam is a betalactam-betalactamase inhibitor which does not penetrate the blood–brain barrier. Therefore, will not be useful to treat bacterial meningitis.
2. Yes, prior receipt of cephalosporin can be a risk factor for extended spectrum betalactamase (ESBL) producing organisms.
3. With the organism showing sensitivity to cefotaxime, one should deescalate from meropenem to cefotaxime and observe the clinical course of the baby closely.
4. 21 days as the clinical picture and CSF is suggestive of meningitis. Switching to oral antibiotics should not be done for treatment of meningitis and treatment should only be by intravenous route.

Case 2

A newborn infant is investigated for unexplained jaundice and hepatomegaly. She is also found to have hydrocephalus, chorioretinitis, and intracranial calcifications.

Questions

1. Which congenital infection would you test for?
2. At what gestation of pregnancy?
   a. The transfer of injection from mother to fetus maximum?
   b. In what trimester fetal infection has the least favorable outcome?.
3. What are the tests to diagnose this infection in the newborn?
4. What is the antibiotic of choice and its duration if newborn is diagnosed to have this infection?

Answers

1. Toxoplasmosis
2. (a) Infection in the last trimester and (b) infection in the first trimester
3. Detection of neonatal IgM and IgA by EIA and/or ISAGA
4. Pyrimethamine plus sulfadiazine for a period of one year.

CASE 3

Interpret the X-ray of a newborn with decreased limb movements and high-grade fever (Fig. 7).

Questions

1. What is the finding on this X-ray ?
2. What is the common causative organism for this infection?
3. What is the common route of transmission of this infection?
4. What is the duration of treatment?

Answers

1. Osteomyelitis of the femur. There is periosteal elevation noted on the femur
2. *Staphylococcus aureus*
3. Hematogenous spread
4. 4–6 weeks.

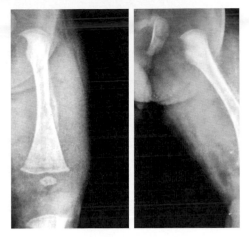

Fig. 7: X-ray limbs of a newborn with decreased limb movements

Case 4

Question

What is the most appropriate antibiotic for the clinical condition in the newborn?

Condition	Name antibiotic
1. Antiretroviral for a newborn born to HIV positive mother for PPTCT	
2. Listeria infection	
3. Prophylaxis against candidemia in ELBW	
4. CMV chorioretinitis and hepatitis	

Answers

1. Nevirapine; 2. Ampicillin; 3. Fluconazole; 4. Ganciclovir.

Case 5

36 hours old male infant is found to be lethargic on routine postnatal rounds. The baby is born at term to a primigravida by normal vaginal delivery. The membranes had ruptured 18 hours before delivery. The mother had fever of 100°F 6 hours prior to delivery. Intravenous cefotaxime was administered to the mother. The baby had fever of 101°F, was feeding well 3 hours before the clinical rounds. He had normal neonatal reflexes. There are no other significant findings.

Question

What would be the best option to manage such a baby?
1. Admit the baby, send CBC, CRP start an antibiotic.
2. Send CBC, CRP, blood culture, and CSF. Start an antibiotic.
3. Keep baby under observation and monitor the clinical course.

Answer: 2

CASE 6

A primigravida delivered a male newborn at term gestation by normal vaginal delivery. On day 5 of life, mother had fever and vesicular rash all over the body.

Questions

1. What is the likely diagnosis?
2. The newborn will almost definitely have varicella (True/False).
3. The greatest risk for severe disease is when maternal varicella occurs 15 days prior to delivery (True/False).
4. The newborn is likely to have congenital varicella syndrome (True/False).
5. Breastfeeding should be continued (True/False).
6. All newborns must be treated with acyclovir (True/False).
7. What are the two options to prevent varicella in this newborn?

Answers

1. Varicella infection
2. False
3. False
4. False
5. True
6. False
7. Options: (a) VZIG 125 units intramuscular, (b) IVIG 400 mg/kg.

Case 7

A 6 days old male, birth weight 3.2 kg, born at term by normal vaginal delivery is admitted for fever 101°F. On examination baby is lethargic, HR 170/min, RR 36/min, CFT 2 sec, anterior fontanel is normal. An intravenous line is established and CBC, CRP, electrolytes and blood cultures are sent. Lumbar puncture is done and CSF samples are sent for routine and culture sensitivity. He is put on cefotaxime and amikacin empirically apart from other routine medications. Total count is 4000/mm³ Platelets 1,03,000/mm³ and CRP is 46 mg/dL, RBS is 40 mg%, electrolytes are normal. CSF routine examination is normal.

On day 3 after admission, the newborn is better, HR is 160/min, RR 36/min RBS 68 mg% and oral feeds are initiated. Blood culture grows *Staphylococcus epidermidis*, sensitive to linezolid and vancomycin.

Questions

Choose the option and give your reason.

1. It is wise to add vancomycin to cefotaxime and amikacin.
2. It is wise to add vancomycin to cefotaxime and stop amikacin.
3. It is wise to add linezolid to cefotaxime and amikacin.
4. None of the above.

Answer

4. *Staphylococcus epidermidis* is a common contaminant. The patient does not have risk factor for this organism like an umbilical catheter. Also baby is showing signs of improvement on the present antibiotics.

CASE 8

A 10 days old newborn, birth weight of 1.4 kg, born at 31 weeks by normal vaginal delivery is transferred to a higher center. The baby was ventilated from day 1 to day 6 for RDS. On examination baby is lethargic, HR 170/min, RR 68/min, CFT 4 secs, SPO_2 84 in room air, MBP is 35 mm Hg, RBS 60 mg%. The anterior fontanel is depressed. There is gross abdominal distension with bilious gastric aspirate. Reports of day 8 are: - total count 2500/mm³, platelets 76000/mm³, CSF examination normal, CRP 74 mg/dL. An X-ray is ordered. Antibiotics used were piperacillin+ tazobactum, amikacin, ceftriaxone, fluconazole, and metronidazole.

Questions

1. What is the likely diagnosis?
2. What are the X-ray features of this disorder?
3. What should be the first step of management strategy of this baby?
4. What should be the starting antibiotic? How should be the antibiotic strategy guided?

Answers

1. Preterm with late onset sepsis with NEC in circulatory failure
2. Supine abdominal X-rays are the mainstay of diagnosis
   If NEC is suspected clinically, or there is concern on supine films, then an additional cross-table lateral or left-lateral decubitus film should be obtained.
   Findings diagnostic of NEC are:
   - Dilated bowel loops (often asymmetrical in distribution)
   - Loss of the normal polygonal gas shape
   - Bowel wall edema with thumb printing
   - Pneumatosis intestinalis (intramural gas)
   - Portal venous gas
   - Pneumoperitoneum secondary to perforation
     » Air on both sides of the bowel (Rigler sign)
     » Air outlining the falciform ligament (football sign)
3. Maintenance of temperature
   - Securing the airway and ventilation
   - Fluid bolus and other supportive care
4. Meropenem and vancomycin since baby is likely to have nosocomial sepsis
   - Reconsider antibiotic choice after culture sensitivity reports are available.

Case 9

A 13-day-old male, birth weight 3.1 kg, born at term by normal vaginal delivery, presents with refusal to feed, lethargy, fever, and convulsion. The baby had cried well immediately after birth. The perinatal period was uneventful. On examination, the baby has generalized tonic-clonic convulsion. The baby is febrile (101°F), HR 180/min, and RR 54/min. There are few vesicular skin lesions over scalp and eyes are sticky.

Questions

1. What is your diagnosis?
2. How you will confirm diagnosis?
3. What is Tzanck test?
4. What are typical forms of presentation of this illness?
5. What is the treatment of this disease?

Answers

1. HSV encephalitis
2. Viral isolation or fluorescent antibody detection from skin and mucocutaneous lesions or DFA, i.e. direct fluorescent antibody from tissues. Viral isolation from oropharynx, nasopharynx, conjunctivae, stool, urine and CSF.
   CSF-PCR
   CT/MRI brain
3. Tzanck test: Cytological examination of vesicular fluid for multinucleated giant cells and intranuclear inclusion with margination of nuclear chromatin.
4. HSV infection in newborn may present as:
   - Skin, eye, and mouth (SEM) infection
   - CNS infection
   - Disseminated infection
5. Drug of choice:
   - Acyclovir 20 mg/kg every 8 hourly
   - Duration for SEM disease—14 days
   - Duration for CNS or disseminated disease—at least 21days, or longer if CSF-PCR remains positive.

MUSCULOSKELETAL

Case 1

A D28, male newborn has decreased movement of right lower limb. He is exclusively breastfed and otherwise well. No other obvious systemic findings are noted. Match the diagnosis with the distinct clinical features.

Question

No	Diagnosis	Feature
1.	Septic arthritis	a. Monoarthritis, absence of fever, well infant
2.	Osteomyelitis	b. Fever, migratory polyarthritis, papulovesicular rash with erythematous base, conjunctival discharge
3.	Reactive arthritis	c. Irritability on handling, maculopapular rash, persistent nasal discharge
4.	Syphilitic arthritis	d. Monoarthritis, rigid range of movements, pain on movement, warmth, no weight bearing
5.	Gonococcemia	e. Symmetric polyarthritis, hepatosplenomegaly
		f. Focal bone tenderness, afebrile, pseudo-paralysis, local swelling, reasonable range of movements

Answer: 1-d, 2-f, 3-a, 4-c, 5-b

Case 2

Questions

Which investigations clinch the diagnosis in a newborn with suspected joint pathology:

No.	Diagnosis	Investigations
1.	Septic arthritis	a. VDRL test of the infant and mother
2.	Osteomyelitis	b. Joint aspiration – synovial fluid analysis
3.	Reactive arthritis	c. X-ray of the affected joint
4.	Syphilitic arthritis	d. Nuclear bone scan
5.	Gonococcemia	e. Diagnosis of exclusion
		f. Gram stain and culture

Answer: 1- b, 2-c, 3-e, 4-a, 5-f

Case 3

This infant is brought for assessment of decreased movement of a limb (Fig. 8). There is no local inflammation.

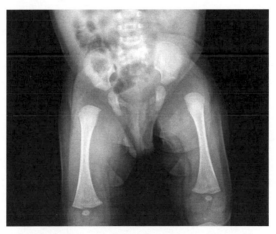

Fig. 8: X-ray of both the joints and femurs

Questions

1. What is the abnormality?
2. Which is the most sensitive test to detect developmental dysplasia (DDH) of hip in first 6 months of life?
3. Name two late clinical manifestations of DDH
4. Barlows and Ortolani test are useful only in first 3 months of life (True or false)
5. What is the treatment of choice in first six months?

Answers

1. Left hip joint is subluxated
2. Ultrasound of hips
3. Limping, toe walking, or a waddling, duck-like gait.....leg length inequality
4. True
5. Closed reduction and immobilization in a Pavlik harness.

Case 4

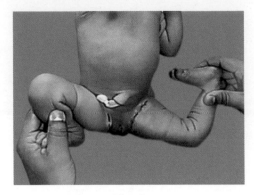

Fig. 9

Questions

1. Identify the condition (Fig. 9).
2. Name the most common condition known to be associated with it.
3. What is the initial treatment of choice?

Answers

1. Congenital dislocation of left knee (Fig. 9)
2. About 50% of patients with congenital knee dislocations will have hip dysplasia affecting one or both hips
3. Reduction with manual manipulation and casting.

Case 5

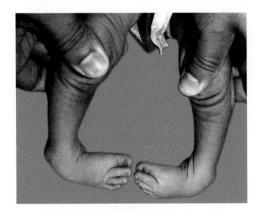

Fig. 10

Questions

1. Identify the problem in this newborn (Fig. 10).
2. Name the four components of the deformity.
3. What is the initial treatment of choice?
4. Name the most common condition known to be associated with it.
5. How early can a prenatal diagnosis be made?

Answers

1. Bilateral club foot

2. Plantar flexion, cavus foot deformity (unusually high arch in the foot), varus (an inversion of the heel that causes the front of the foot to turn inward) and adduction of forefoot.
3. Stretching and casting (Ponseti method)
4. Spina bifida
5. 18–21 weeks.

Case 6

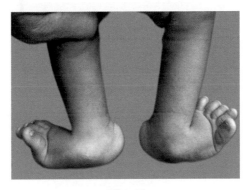

Fig. 11

Questions

1. Identify (Fig. 11).
2. What is the underlying anatomical problem?
3. Name the two most common disorders associated with it.
4. What is the initial treatment of choice?

Answers

1. Congenital vertical talus (Rockerbottom foot)
2. Rigid, irreducible talonavicular dislocation
3. About 50% associated with a neuromuscular (myelodysplasia, arthrogryposis, diastematomyelia) or genetic disorder
4. Serial manipulation and casting for three months.

Case 7

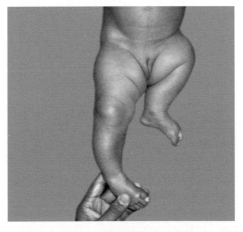

Fig. 12

Questions

1. Identify the problem in this newborn (Fig. 12).
2. What is the most common associated deformity?
3. What is the basis to consider lengthening or prosthesis?
4. At what age are treatment options initiated?

Answers

1. Proximal femoral focal deficiency
2. Congenital fibular hemimelia (50%–80%)
3. A predicted limb discrepancy at maturity not exceeding 20 cm is an indication for lengthening. Otherwise prosthesis should be considered.
4. Three years of age.

Case 8

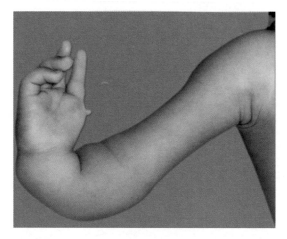

Fig. 13

Questions

1. Identify the problem in the newborn (Fig. 13).
2. Name two hematologic abnormalities associated with it.
3. What anomalies do you search for in such an infant?

Answers

1. Radial hemimelia (a congenital longitudinal deficiency of the radius bone of the forearm characterized by partial or total absence of the radius).
2. Thrombocytopenia (TAR syndrome) and anemia (Fanconi's anemia)
3. VACTERL (vertebral, anal, cardiac, tracheaesophagial, renal, limb anamolies).

JAUNDICE

Case 1

A Baby male was born at 35+6 weeks by normal vaginal delivery to a 22-year-old primigravida mother because of spontaneous onset of labor. Mother's blood group was O+ve and she had gestational diabetes. No risk factors for sepsis. Baby was born with birth weight of 2.1 kg, cried immediately after birth, feeding well and was discharged after 48 hours. He was brought to the emergency department at 80 hours of life with parental concerns – "looks very yellow since yesterday but is alert".

Questions

1. How will you do early risk assessment (triage management) of this neonate?
2. What are the important clinical risk factors in the history you would like to highlight to predict severe jaundice while evaluating this neonate?

Answers

1. The trial management of this newborn would include:

- Rapid clinical examination to check
  - » Severity of jaundice
  - » TcB test
  - » Neurologic examination for muscle tone, behavior, and cry pattern.
- Plot TcB and recent TSB level on the AAP bilirubin nomogram for risk assessment and for exchange transfusion.
- Weigh against the potential risk of ABE and timeliness/safety of interventions (experience is essential).
- Communicate with families regarding potential of imminent risk.

2. Major

- What was the predischarge TSB/TcB(>95th percentile)
- Any blood group incompatibility
- Gestational age 35–36 weeks and LBW
- Any sibling received phototherapy
- Cephalohematoma or significant bruising during perinatal transition
- Exclusive but suboptimalbreast-feeding
- Early onset sepsis

Case 2

A 3-day-old male term neonate referred to you from periphery with severe jaundice, SBR 35 mg/dL. He was born by normal vaginal delivery to a primigravida mother. He cried immediately after birth. His birth weight was 3.2 kg. Mother's blood group was AB positive. There was difficulty in establishing feeding. He has passed urine twice in last 24 hours. On admission to ER he weighed 2.7 kg. He is very irritable, had 1episode of seizure on day 2 and not accepting oral feeds.

Questions

1. What is the probable diagnosis?
2. What are the risk factors for severe Jaundice in term neonate?
3. What are the four preliminary things which you would like to do in the emergency management of the baby-"crash cart approach"?
4. Enumerate 5 important investigations which you would like to send urgently.

Answers

1. Severe hyperbilirubinemia with acute bilirubin encephalopathy with possible dyslectrolytemia
2. **Risk factors are:**
   - Jaundice within first 24 hours of life
   - Unrecognized hemolysis like ABO or Rh incompatability
   - G6PD deficiency
   - Sibling with history of severe hyperbilirubinemia
   - Nonoptimal sucking or nursing
   - Infection
   - Cephalhematoma or bruising
3. **For preliminary things to do:**
   - Assess the sick neonate for airway, breathing and circulation and shift the baby to NICU immediately.
   - Start intensive phototherapy as early as possible.
   - Establish an IV/central access urgently and arrange blood for double volume exchange transfusion.
   - Consider immune globulin (IVIG) for isoimmune hemolytic disease.
4. **Laboratory tests (do not wait for results to start treatment):**
   - Repeat TSB and direct bilirubin level
   - Serum albumin, serum electrolytes
   - Blood type (ABO, Rh)
   - Direct antibody test (Coombs')
   - CBC, differential and smear for cell morphology; reticulocyte count
   - G6PD enzyme assay (quantitative)
   - Urine for reducing substances and other tests: as needed.

Case 3

G2P1 mother with blood group O-ve was taken up for emergency LSCS. She did not receive Anti-D in first pregnancy. The fetus had signs of hydrops at 30 weeks of gestation. After covering for antenatal steroids, an in utero tranfusion was performed. At 35 weeks of gestation, there was evidence of increase MCA blood flow and early signs of hydrops.

Questions

1. As a neonatologist what delivery room preparation you would like to ensure?
2. What are the indications of exchange transfusion in this neonate?
3. What is the role of IVIG in this situation and in what dosage it should be administered?

Answers

1. Delivery room management: At delivery, assessment includes evaluation of the infant's respiratory and cardiovascular system, and the severity of hemolysis. Pallor, tachycardia, and tachypnea are findings suggestive of symptomatic anemia. Respiratory distress may also be due to pleural effusions or pulmonary hypoplasia in infants with hydrops fetalis.

In all cases if HDFN is suspected or known, cord blood should be sent for the following:
- Blood type and antiglobulin (Coombs) test to confirm the diagnosis.
- Hematocrit, reticulocyte count, and bilirubin concentration to guide decisions on therapeutic interventions (e.g. transfusions and/or phototherapy).
- Cross match for subsequent transfusion.

2. **Indications for exchange transfusion**
   - A cord bilirubin level greater than 5 mg/dL (77 mmol/L) has been suggested as an initial threshold for exchange transfusion. However, the child should be started on intensive phototherapy and serial rise in the TSB should be monitored. A rise of TSB greater than 0.5 mg/dL (8 mmol/L) per hour, despite intensive phototherapy, as an indication for exchange transfusion.
   - Signs of acute bilirubin encephalopathy as hypotonia, irritability, shrill cry, poor suck or seizures.

3. **Immune globulin therapy**: AAP guidelines recommends the administration of IVIG in infants with HDFN if the TSB is rising despite intensive phototherapy or is within 2 or 3 mg/dL (34–51 mmol/L) of the threshold for exchange transfusion. The recommended dose is 500–1000 mg/kg given over two hours, and the dose may be repeated in 12 hours if necessary.

Case 4

Questions

1. **Identify the nomogram (Fig. 14A). What do the shaded areas depict?**

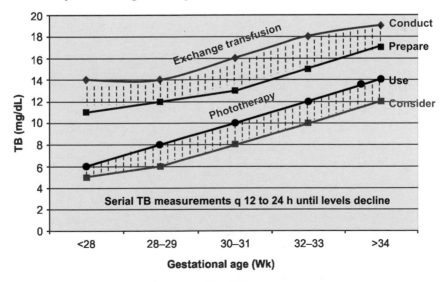

Fig. 14A

2. Identify the figure (Fig. 14B).

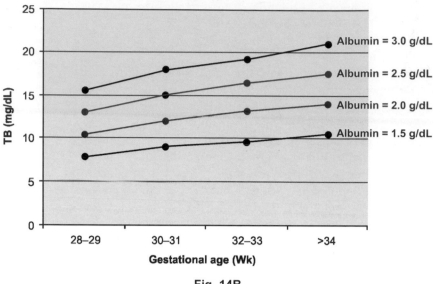

Fig. 14B

3. What is BAMR?

4. What are the limitations of BAMR?

Answers

1. Maisels charts suggesting use of phototherapy and exchange transfusion in preterm infants less than 35 weeks GA.
   The shaded bands represent the degree of uncertainty and provides time for consider and prepare for early phototherapy and exchange transfusion respectively.
2. Recommended use of BAMR for initiation of exchange transfusions (BAMR values have been calculated to bilirubin (mg/dL)/albumin (g/dL). Values above the thresholds for select serum albumin values of 1.5, 2.0, 2.5, and 3.0 g/dL are presented as bands above which bilirubin is likely to be displaced and may be neurotoxic).
3. Bilirubin albumin molar ratio (BAMR). The BAMR may serve as an approximate surrogate for unconjugated bilirubin levels, and can be used as an additional factor in determining the need for exchange transfusion in neonates of 35 or more weeks GA. Preterm infants are likely to have lower serum albumin levels, and it has been suggested that the BAMR would be a good measure of the risk for bilirubin toxicity based on birth weight.
4. Factors (e.g. acidosis, use of multiple drugs, elevated free fatty acids, and bilirubin photoisomers) in preterm neonates may interfere with bilirubin–albumin binding or binding of bilirubin to sites other than albumin.

Case 5

An extreme preterm (birth weight of 750 grams and gestation of 26 weeks) at 3 weeks of age is being treated for PDA, NEC stage II and hypoglycemia. The newborn is on CPAP and had received TPN and blood products in the recent past. On examination, the newborn has pallor and jaundice.

Questions

1. Enumerate four probable causes for jaundice in this newborn.
2. Name four tests in order of priority you would do in this case.

Answers

1. **Differentials**
   - New episode of sepsis (gram-negative)
   - Prolonged TPN using intralipids-leading to cholestasis
   - Multiple transfusions- probable CMV hepatitis
   - Multiple antibioticsfor sepsis
   - Intraventricular hemorrhage.
2. **Investigations**
   - Complete blood picture, CRP, blood culture for sepsis
   - Urine examination and urine culture
   - Stop TPN and send liver function tests, direct and indirect bilirubin levels complete lipid profile and triglyceride levels.
   - CMV IgM
   - Scans- NSG and USG abdomen to look for liver echotexture and any thrombus in major blood vessels.

Case 6

Questions

1. What is the tetrad of kernicterus?
2. Which areas of the brain have specific predilection for BIND?

Answers

1. **Term kernicterus should be reserved for chronic sequele of acute bilirubin encephalopathy. Clinical signs include:**
   - Motor—choreoathetoid cerebral palsy, motor delay
   - Cochlear—sensorineural deafness
   - Oculomotor—Gaze abnormalities, upward gaze paresis
   - Dental enamel dysplasia.
2. **The most common affected areas are:**
   - Basal ganglia, particularly globus pallidus and subthalamic nuclei
   - Hippocampus, specifically sectors H2–3
   - Substantia nigra
   - Cranial nerve nuclei–occulomotor, vestibular, cochlear and facial
   - Reticular formation of pons
   - Inferior olivary nucleus
   - Cerebellar nuclei, especially the dentate
   - Anterior horn cell of spinal cord.

Case 7

Questions

1. What are the common drugs that displace bilirubin from albumin-binding sites? (any 5)
2. At what serum albumin value there should be a concern for bilirubin toxicity?

Answers

1. Ceftriaxone, sulfisoxazole, cefmetazole, sulfamethoxazole, cefonicid, cefotetan, and salicylates.
2. One molecule of albumin binds with one molecule of bilirubin, giving potential equimolar B:A ratio. If B:A ratio increase 0.8, chances of free bilirubin molecule is there in blood. Molar ratio <0.65 is considered safe in term and late preterm (5.5 mg of bilirubin per gram of albumin).

Case 8

A preterm infant (34 weeks at birth) is examined for new onset jaundice. The newborn had RDS, probable sepsis in the immediate neonatal period. The infant had received TPN for the first 7 days of life. The blood reports indicate TSB of 5 mg/dL, direct bilirubin of 3.8 mg/dL, SGOT of 650 U/L, SGPT of 120 U/L, ALT 138 U/L and GGT of 1200 U/L.

Questions

1. What is the provisional diagnosis?
2. Name four tests in priority that you would do.

Answer

1. Infantile cholestasis with disproportionately elevated serum GGT and ALP, suggesting biliary disease.
2. Should be investigated on following lines:
   - Blood – CBP, Blood culture, liver function test, coagulation profile and free T4 TSH.
   - Urine – complete urine examination and cultures
   - Abdominal USG
   - HIDA scan.

Case 9

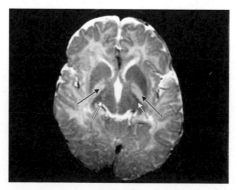

Fig. 15

Questions

1. Identify the image (Fig. 15).
2. Write three differentials.

Answers

1. Axial T2-weighted MR image of the brain showing increased T2 signal in the globus pallidus bilaterally (black arrows) and minimally increased signal in the subthalamic nuclei (white arrows).
2. The three differentials are:
   - Acute bilirubin encephalopathy
   - Mitochondrial disorders
   - Pyruvate dehydrogenase deficiency.

Case 10

Questions

1. **Enumerate three criteria for effective phototherapy.**
2. **Name 3 factors which affect the efficacy of phototherapy?**

Answer

1. Criteria for phototherapy:
   - Specific light wavelength at specific narrow peak (460 nm, blue)
   - The narrow bandwidth delivered at an irradiance (dose) of $\geq 25\text{-}30$ uW/ cm^2/nm (measured specifically for the selected light wavelength).
   - It should be exposed to at least 80% of body surface area

2. Efficacy of phototherapy:
   - Minimum distance between the device and patient such that footprint of the light covers maximum surface area with minimum physical barriers.
   - Patient factors like severity of jaundice, surface area proportions, dermal thickness, pigmentation and skin perfusion.
   - Duration of treatment to specific bilirubin threshold.

INBORN ERRORS OF METABOLISM

Case 1

A term baby presents on day 7 of life with poor feeding, vomiting and decreased activity. Antenatal period was uncomplicated. The baby was born by normal vaginal delivery and was exclusively breastfeed. On examination, the newborn had muscle rigidity, opisthotonus and episodes of hypertonicity alternating with flaccidity. Laboratory data reveal hypoglycemia, metabolic acidosis, and cerebral edema. Plasma levels of leucine, isoleucine, and valine are elevated.

Questions

1. What is the most probable diagnosis?
2. What is the mode of inheritance?
3. What is the mainstay of treatment?
4. Which vitamin therapy trial may be attempted?

Answers

1. MSUD
2. Autosomal recessive
3. Formula feed-protein restrictive. Dietary restriction of branched-chain amino acids
4. Thiamine.

Case 2

Questions

Eye examination gives clues to the diagnosis of IEM. Match the eye finding with the IEM.

Eye sign	IEM
1. Lenticular cataract	a. Tay–Sachs disease
2. Dislocated lens	b. Peroxisomal disorders
3. Retinitis pigmentosa	c. Homocystinuria
4. Cherry red macular spot	d. Methylmalonic acidemia
	e. Galactosemia

Answers: 1-e, 2-c, 3-b, 4-a

Case 3

Questions

You are evaluating a day 4, preterm newborn with persistent hypoglycemia. You run a battery of tests to identify the underlying cause. How do you interpret A, B, C, D, and E in the Flowchart 1?

Flowchart 1

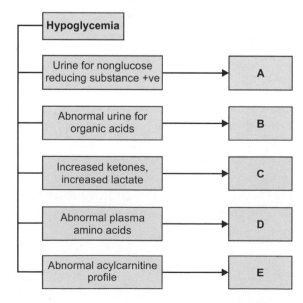

Answers

A. Galactosemia, hereditary fructose intolerance, tyrosinemia type 1
B. Organic academia
C. GSD type 1
D. Disorders of amino acid metabolism
E. Fatty acid oxidation defects.

Case 4

An infant presents at 6 weeks of age with feeding difficulty, vomiting and reduced tone. During the last week she developed an erythematous exfoliative generalized rash and partial alopecia. Laboratory data reveal metabolic acidosis, ketosis, and hyperammonemia.

Questions

1. What is the most probable diagnosis?
2. What is the mode of inheritance?
3. Which vitamin therapy is most beneficial?
4. What CT brain findings are suggestive of this disorder?

Answers

1. Multiple carboxylase deficiency (biotinidase deficiency)
2. Autosomal recessive
3. Biotin
4. Bilateral basal ganglia calcifications.

Case 5

Question

Match the treatment option with the IEM disorder

Disorder	Treatment option
1. Maple syrup urine disease	a. Sodium phenylbutyrate
2. Methylmalonic acidemia	b. Carnitine
3. Urea cycle disorder	c. Glycine
4. Isovaleric acidemia	d. Thiamine
5. Organic acidemia	e. Vitamin B_{12}
6. Multiple carboxylase deficiency	f. Biotin
7. Homocystinuria	g. Pyridoxine
	h. Vitamin A

Answers: 1-d, 2-e, 3-a, 4-c, 5-b, 6-f, 7-g

CASE 6

Question

You are reviewing the diagnosis of an IEM disorder. Match the following

Metabolic error	Diagnosis
1. Phenylketonuria	a. Branched-chain a-keto acid dehydrogenase deficiency
2. GSD Type la	b. β-glucocerebrosidase deficiency
3. Zellweger syndrome	c. α-galactosidase A deficiency
4. Gaucher's disease	d. Peroxisome membrane protein
5. Galactosemia	e. Galactose 1-phosphate uridyltransferase deficiency
6. Maple syrup urine disease	f. Glucose-6-phosphatase deficiency
	g. Phenylalanine hydroxylase deficiency

Answers: 1-g, 2-f, 3-d, 4-b, 5-e, 6-a

Case 7

Questions

You are reviewing a term newborn on day 3 of life for a suspected IEM. You identify there is hyperammonemia. You run a battery of tests to Identify the underlying cause. How do you interpret A, B, C, and D in the Flowchart 2:

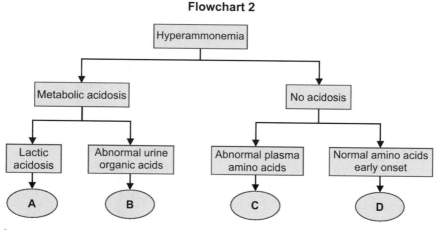

Flowchart 2

Answers

A. Pyruvate metabolic defects, mitochondrial defects
B. Organic acidemia
C. Urea cycle defect
D. Transient hyperammonemia of newborn.

Case 8

Questions

You are evaluating a term newborn on day 3 of life for suspected IEM. You identify metabolic acidosis. You run a battery of tests to identify the underlying cause. How do you interpret A, B, C, and D the Flowchart 3?

Answers

A. GSD 1, hereditary fructose intolerance
B. Pyruvate metabolism defects
C. Mitochondrial defects, pyruvate carboxylase deficiency.
D. Organic academia, FAO defects.

Flowchart 3

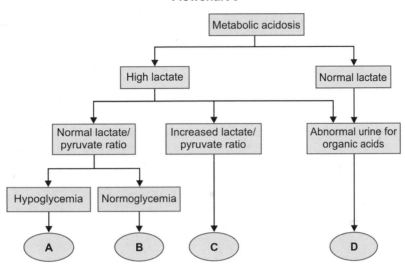

Case 9

A newborn presents on day 3 of life with poor feeding, vomiting, and lethargy. He becomes nonresponsive within few hours of hospitalization. ABG shows respiratory alkalosis. Hyperammonemia is noted. The urine orotic acid level is also elevated.

Questions

1. What is the most probable diagnosis?
2. What is the mode of inheritance?
3. What medications should be immediately initiated for the present crisis?
4. What marks the prognosis for this infant?

Answers

1. Ornithine transcarbamylase deficiency
2. X-linked
3. Protein free 24 hours, IV arginine and a combination of sodium benzoate and sodium phenylacetate
4. Duration of coma, not severity of hyperammonemia.

Case 10

A term infant is admitted to the hospital on day 7 with lethargy, fever, and increasing jaundice. You notice firm hepatomegaly. Blood glucose on admission is 10 mg/dL, total and direct bilirubin values are 15 and 7 mg/dL, respectively, and liver enzymes are AST700

units/L, and ALT, 650 units/L. After 30 hours the blood culture isolates a Gram-negative rod.

Questions

1. What is the most probable diagnosis?
2. What is the mode of inheritance?
3. What bedside investigation that gives a clue to the diagnosis?
4. What is the treatment of choice?

Answers

1. Galactosemia
2. Autosomal recessive
3. Urine for glucose-nonglucose reducing substances
4. Galactose free diet.

Case 11

A male infant presents on day 8 of life with vomiting and poor oral intake. On admission, he is noticed to be hypotonia and is unresponsive to stimuli. Laboratory findings reveal 4+ ketonuria; arterial blood gas, pH 6.7; PCO_2, 20 mm Hg; PO_2, 85 mm Hg; anion gap, 36 mEq/L

Questions

1. What is the most probable diagnosis?
2. What is the mode of inheritance?
3. What vitamin therapy may be beneficial?

Answers

1. Methylmalonic academia
2. AR
3. B_{12}

NUTRITION AND GROWTH

Questions

1. Name the major whey protein in breast milk.
2. Name three specific immune-active proteins in breast milk.
3. Name two essential fatty acids present in breast milk.
4. For breastfed infants, which nutrient supplementation is necessary in preterm and term neonates? Also mention their doses.

Answers

1. α-lactalbumin
2. Lactoferrin, lysozyme, and secretory immunoglobulin A (sIgA)
3. Linoleic acid and linolenic acid
4. Preterm babies:
   - Calcium: 120–140 mg/kg/day
   - Phosphorus: 60–90 mg/kg/day
   - Iron: 2–3 mg/kg elemental iron

- Vitamin D: 400–800 IU/day
- Multivitamins

Term babies:
- Vitamin D – 400–800 IU/day
- Iron: 2–3 mg/kg at 4 months of age.

Questions

Below are important electrolytes and minerals in breast milk; match the mineral/electrolyte with its breast milk content (mg per liter):

a. Calcium   1. 120 – 250
b. Phosphorus   2. 200 – 250
c. Iron   3. 120 – 140
d. Sodium   4. 400 – 550
e. Potassium   5. 0.3 – 0.9

Answers: a. 2; b. 3; c. 5; d. 1; e. 4

Questions

Match the following breast milk component with its function in human body.

a. Lactoferrin   1. Antioxidants
b. Epidermal growth factor 2. Anti-inflammatory, epithelial barrier function
c. Glutathione peroxidase   3. Prevents lipid oxidation
d. Vitamin A, E, C   4. Immunomodulation
e. Cytokines   5. Luminal surveillance and intestinal repair

Answers: a. 4; b. 5; c. 3; d. 1; e. 2

Questions

1. Mention three indications for parenteral nutrition.
2. What is the maximum dose of dextrose, amino acids and lipids in a preterm neonate?
3. Which trace element is added on Day 1 of TPN?
4. List the management strategies for PN related cholestasis?
5. Which complication is likely to occur due to use of glass bottles for TPN?

Answers

1. Babies <1000 g, NEC, congenital anomalies of GIT
2. 18 g/kg/day of glucose; 4.5 g/kg/day of amino acids and 3 grams/kg/day of lipid.
3. Zinc
4. Stop/modify TPN, early initiation of enteral feeds, fish-oil based TPN.
5. Aluminum toxicity.

Questions

1. What is the chart shown in Figure 16? Is it a growth standard or reference?
2. What growth chart is used for preterm babies beyond term gestation? Till what postnatal age will you use corrected age for growth charting?
3. Which are the acceptable growth targets for weight, length and head circumference in preterm growing babies?
4. Which age group is covered by INTERGROWTH 21st growth chart?

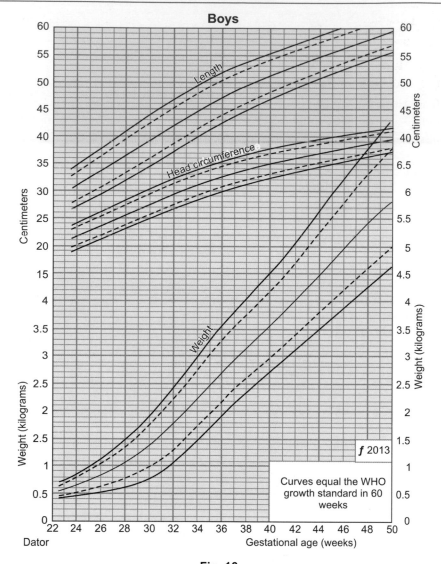

Fig. 16:

Answers

1. Modified Fenton growth chart; Reference growth chart
2. WHO growth chart; Corrected 40 weeks
3. Weight velocity: 15 g/kg/day,
   Length velocity: 0.75 cm/week,
   Head circumference velocity: 0.75 cm/week
4. 32 weeks to 64 weeks

Case 1

20-days-old baby with a birth weight of 1.5 kg is brought to the follow-up clinic with a weight of 1.4 Kg. Baby is on spoon feeds and

is taking 20 mL of breast milk, 10 times a day. Otherwise baby is well on examination.

Questions
1. Calculate energy and protein intake of this baby?
2. What is the recommended daily enteral energy and protein intake in preterm babies?
3. What intervention will you take to improve the growth for this baby?

Answers
1. Energy: 89 kcal/kg/day; 1.5 g/kg/day
2. Energy: 110–135 kcal/kg/day. Protein: 3.5–4 grams/kg/day
3. Increase feed volume to 200 mL/kg/day; Add HMF to feeds Kangaroo mother care, reduce thermal stress.

NEPHROLOGY

Case 1

A day-2-old neonate presented with dribbling micturition, abdominal distention. Below is the investigation.

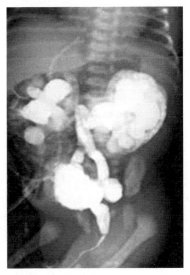

Fig. 17

Questions
1. What is the investigation (Fig. 17)?
2. What is the diagnosis?
3. What are the findings on X-ray?
4. How do you treat this problem?
5. What are the long-term complications?

Answers
1. Micturating cystourethrogram
2. Posterior urethral valve

3. Dilated posterior urethra, vesicoureteral reflux, trabeculation over bladder, diverticula.
4. Rule out urine infection, look for acidosis and electrolyte imbalances, cystoscopy and valve fulguration/ablation.
5. Repeated urinary tract infection, persistent vesicoureteral reflux, valve bladder syndrome, chronic kidney disease.

Case 2

A 34 week, 1.4 kg, male newborn is born to a mother with severe oligohydramnios. The newborn is noted to have clubbed foot, flat facies and broad nasal bridge.

Questions

1. What is the condition?
2. What are the possible underlying renal diseases?
3. What is immediate risk for this newborn?
4. What determines the long-term outcome if the newborn survives immediate risk?

Answers

1. Potter's syndrome/sequence
2. Bilateral renal agenesis, obstructive uropathies, bilateral cystic kidney disease, bilateral renal hypoplasia.
3. Respiratory distress due to pulmonary hypoplasia
4. Renal function.

Case 3

A day 14 active and playful neonate, presented with oliguria, abdominal distention and generalized edema. At birth the newborn weighed 2.9 kg, had history of polyhydraminos and large placenta. He is born to parents of 3rd degree consanguineous marriage. Previous sibling died of kidney disease in infancy.

Questions

1. What is the diagnosis?
2. What gene mutations are associated with this diagnosis?
3. What is the treatment?
4. Which endocrine disorder is associated with this condition?

Answers

1. Congenital nephrotic syndrome
2. NPHS1, NPHS2, WT1
3. Good nutrition, control edema, preventing thrombosis and infections. Prepare the family for kidney transplant (no role of steroid).
4. Hypothyroidism.

Case 4

A Full-term newborn male newborn with a birth weight of 3.1 kg is admitted to the NICU. Fetal ultrasound at 28 weeks had revealed a unilateral hydronephrosis.

Questions

1. What clinical examination should be done in this newborn?
2. When shall we plan ultrasound of the kidneys and why?
3. What are the common conditions that present with unilateral fetal hydronephrosis?

Answers

1. Palpable bladder, palpable kidneys, genital examination and urine stream.
2. Abdominal sonography should be after 72 hours, as a scan done before may miss a mild hydronephrosis due to physiological oliguria.
3. Vesicoureteral reflux, pelvicureteric junction obstruction, vesicoureteral junction obstruction.

Case 5

A day 3 neonate born by spontaneous vaginal delivery presented with no urine output for 2 days

Questions

1. What is the relevant history for this newborn?
2. What relevant exam is required in this newborn?

Answers

1. The relevant history would include:
   - Antenatal sonography showing oligohydramnios, kidney anomalies
   - Maternal drug history
   - Birth asphyxia
   - Has infant ever voided
   - Was feeding adequate.
2. The relevant examination should include:
   - Present weight (weight loss or gain)
   - Temperature, pulses, CRT, BP, signs of dehydration
   - Edema, hypertension, ascites, congestive cardiac failure
   - Enlarged bladder, enlarged kidneys.

Case 6

A day 7 neonate of birth weight of 3.2 kg presented with palpable abdominal mass. USG abdomen showed right kidney 5.2 × 1.8 cm, multiple cysts, echogenic intervening renal parenchyma and left kidney of normal echogenicity and size 3.8 × 1.9 cm.

Questions
1. What is the diagnosis
2. How do you council the parents of this newborn?
3. Which investigation will make the diagnosis clear?

Answers
1. Multicystic dysplastic kidney on right side
2. Right kidney is nonfunctional, with age it generally undergo auto-nephrectomy, rarely requires surgical intervention. Left kidney is normal. One normal kidney is sufficient for life.
3. DMSA scan.

Case 7

In a sonography done for oligohydramnios, the fetal kidneys were normal in shape but markedly enlarged and diffusely echogenic.

Questions
1. What is the most probable diagnosis?
2. What is the most common associated anomaly with this condition?
3. What is renal outcome of this patient?

Answers
1. Autosomal recessive polycystic kidney disease
2. Hepatic fibrosis
3. Most of them progress to end stage renal disease (ESRD) within 1st decade.

Case 8

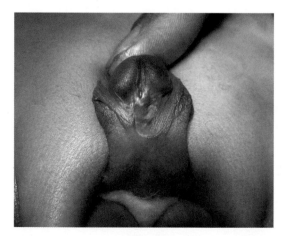

Fig. 18

Questions
1. Identify the condition in this photograph (Fig. 18).
2. Classify this clinical condition?
3. What are the associated anomalies with this condition?
4. What instructions should be given to a neonate regarding circumcision?

Answers

1. Hypospadias
2. The types of hypospadias are anterior or distal, middle or mid-penile and posterior or proximal
3. Undescended testis, inguinal hernia, bifid scrotum
4. Circumcision should not be done before correction of hypospadiasis.

EMERGENCY AND CRITICAL CARE

Case 1

A full term 3.4 kg baby, born after a spontaneous vaginal delivery, is noted to have pink lips and dusky soles. Antenatal and delivery events were uncomplicated. The baby is alert and active, breathing is regular and saturation in the right upper limb is 95%.

Questions

1. What is the cause of duskiness in the baby?
2. What is the most likely cause?
3. What is the best action you will take?
4. Why is right upper limb preferred for detecting oxygen status in the first hour of life?

Answers

1. Acrocyanosis
2. Cold stress
3. Ensure warmth: Skin to skin contact, keep room warm, cover the baby.
4. Measurements are obtained fastest from the right hand probably owing to better perfusion, higher blood pressure and oxygenation in preductal vessels.

Case 2

An infant is brought to the hospital at 3 weeks of age for difficulty in breathing and feeding. On examination HR is 180/min, RR is 72/min, rectal temperature is 37.4°C, BP is 80/50 mm of Hg and had hepatomegaly with a liver 4 cm below the costal margin. Sepsis screen is negative.

Questions

1. What is the most likely diagnosis?
2. Name two cardiac disorders presenting without murmur.
3. Which cardiac disorders that deteriorate on oxygen therapy?
4. Which is the preferred mode of administration of digoxin.

Answers

1. Congestive cardiac failure
2. Left to right shunt with CCF (murmur reappears once stabilized), TGA with a balanced shunt, coarctation of aorta, cortriatrium, cardiomyopathy, arrhythmia, and myocarditis.

3. Duct dependent
4. Oral.

Case 3

A female baby with an uneventful pregnancy and delivery is brought to the emergency for decreased activity on day 20 of life. There are no localizing signs on examination. Fundus reveals bilateral and multiple retinal hemorrhages.

Questions

1. What is the most probable diagnosis?
2. What systemic survey should you order next?
3. Name the most common intracranial lesion associated?
4. Name a metabolic disorder that mimics this condition?

Answers

1. Child abuse
2. Skeletal: The skeletal survey is positive in 60% of cases involving non-accidental injury.
3. Subdural hemorrhage
4. Glutaric aciduria type 1.

Case 4

You are called to evaluate a 3.5-kg female newborn delivered by an elective cesarean section. The staff nurse noted that the baby to be grunting at 10 minutes of age. By the time you see the temperature is 37°C, respiratory rate is 65/min, mild chest in-drawings, occasional grunt, HR is 145/min, saturation is 95%, and the child is vigorous.

Questions

1. What is the most probable diagnosis?
2. Name two maternal morbidities that predispose to this condition.
3. What is the usual time required for the resolution of this condition?
4. Name two classical radiological findings of his condition.

Answers

1. Transient tachypnea of newborn
2. Diabetes, asthma
3. Within 48–72 hours after birth
4. Good volume lungs, prominent perihilar vascular markings, transverse fissure, mild cardiomegaly.

Case 5

A large-for-gestational-age infant with a birth weight of 4,500-g is admitted on day 5 of life with jaundice and total serum bilirubin level of 21 mg/dL. The infant appears vigorous. There is no anemia or polycythemia, but on examination has a large cephalhematoma. The baby is exclusively breastfed and maternal blood group is A, Rh +ve

Questions

1. What is the best treatment for cephalhematoma?
2. What is intensive phototherapy?
3. Name two set of infants in whom AAP charts for jaundice management does not apply.
4. What are the risk factors that define the curves on AAP phototherapy charts?

Answers

1. No intervention
2. Giving phototherapy with an irradiance of atleast 30 $\mu W/cm^2/nm$
3. <34 w, >7 d old, <24 h old
4. Gestation, hemolysis, G6PD, asphyxia, low albumin, sepsis, acidosis, temperature instability and lethargy.

Case 6

A 2-week-old infant is brought to the emergency room with lethargy following two episodes of frank large blood stained vomitus. He is noted have severe pallor. He was born at home and was on exclusive breastfeeding from birth. There are no specific findings on systemic examination.

Questions

1. What is the most probable diagnosis?
2. What tests confirms the clinical suspicion?
3. What preventive measure could have prevented this tragedy?
4. What is the first drug of choice for treatment?

Answers

1. Hemorrhagic disease of newborn (HDN/VKDB)
2. PT, PTT prolonged but normal fibrinogen and d-dimers
3. Vitamin K at birth
4. Vitamin K.

Case 7

A 3.4 kg, term, breastfed, the baby is noted to have persistent hyperbilirubinemia at 2 week of age. On physical examination, the infant is found to mottled skin, decreased tone, an umbilical hernia, and an anterior fontanel measuring 4 6 cm.

Questions

1. What is the most probable clinical diagnosis?
2. What bedside clues rule out conjugated hyperbilirubinemia?
3. Name the confirmatory test.
4. How do you confirm breast milk jaundice?

Answers

1. Congenital hypothyroidism.
2. Absence of high colored urine and clay colored stools.
3. T3, T4, TSH.
4. It is a diagnosis of exclusion.

NECROTIZING ENTEROCOLITIS

Case1

Questions

Bell's Stages of Necrotizing Enterocolitis: Fill in the blanks

1. Stage I: Suspected NEC
    - IA: Apnea, abdominal distention, gastric residue
    - IB: Stage IA with_____
2. Stage II: Definite NEC
    - IIA: Mild illness, radiology shows pathognomic sign:_____
    - IIB: Moderate illness, metabolic acidosis, portal venous gas, ascites
3. Stage III: Advanced NEC
    - Stage IIIa: Severe NEC with intact bowel
    - Stage IIIb: Severe NEC with _____

Answers

1. Gross blood in stool.
2. Pneumatosis intestinalis.
3. Perforation.

Case 2

Questions

Mark true or false for the following statements regarding NEC

1. In term infants NEC occurs at an earlier age than preterm.
2. Ranitidine in preterm increases risk of NEC.
3. Antenatal steroids increases risk of NEC.

Answers

1. True.
2. True.
3. False.

Case 3

Questions

Mark the correct statement on NEC.

1. Triad of NEC consist of all *except* following:
    - Thrombocytopenia
    - Hyponatremia
    - Hypernatremia
    - Blood in stool.
2. Risk factors for NEC all *except*:
    - Prematurity
    - Birth-asphyxia
    - PDA
    - Placental insufficiency
    - Antenatal steroids
    - Blood transfusions.

3. Pnematosis intestinalis is seen in all of the following *except*:
   - Infectious enteritis
   - Necrotizing enterocolitis
   - Meconium ileus
   - Steroid use.
4. Which is considered as poorest prognosis sign in NEC among following?
   - Pnematosis intestinalis
   - Persistent thrombocytopenia
   - Portal gas
   - Metabolic acidosis
   - Blood in stool.
5. Etiological factors suggested in NEC are all *except*:
   - Indomethacin
   - Formula feeds
   - Trophic feeds
   - Rapid advancement of feeds
   - Vitamin E.

Answers

a-3; b-5; c-4; d-3; e-3

Case 4

26 week preterm baby delivered by normal vaginal delivery with respiratory distress syndrome was admitted in NICU. Baby received two doses of surfactant and was ventilated for four days. Baby was started on breast milk through nasogastric tube on day 3, was tolerating well, feeds slowly increased to 10 mL every 2 hourly. On day 12 baby developed abdominal distension and increased gastric aspirates. X-ray of the abdomen is shown in Figs 19A and B.

Questions

1. Identify two radiological findings (arrows).
2. What is the diagnosis and the staging?
3. In Figure 19B, the X-ray repeated after 48 hours, what is the finding and the stage?
4. What is the treatment if the newborn is very sick and has multiorgan dysfunction?

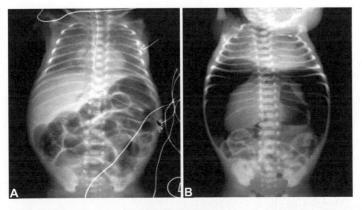

Figs 19A and B

Answers

1. Portal venous gas and pneumatosis intestinalis
2. Necrotizing enterocolitis and stage II
3. Pneumoperitoneum, stage III B
4. Paracentesis and supportive management.

Case 5

A 6-hour-old female neonate is brought to the emergency department with birth weight of 1 kg. The baby was born to a multigravida mother with previous two first trimester spontaneous abortions at 32 weeks of gestation by emergency LSCS. The indication for LSCS was abnormal Doppler flow in the umbilical arteries.

On Examination

Head circumference is 26 cm; length is 33 cm; heart rate is 154/min; respiratory rate is 50/min; temperature is 36.8°C; peripheries warm and pink. There were many bluish purple palpable nodules all over the skin, on cardiac evaluation systolic murmur was heard in the left infraclavicular area. Per abdomen examination revealed enlarged liver and spleen.

Questions

1. When will you start feed in these neonates?
2. Classify the IUGR in this neonate.
3. What are the causes for this type of IUGR?

Answers

1. As the neonate is having history of abnormal Doppler in utero, feeds to be differed till 24-48 hours as these infants are at high risk of feed intolerance and necrotizing enterocolitis.
2. As head circumference, length and weight are equally affected and ponderal index is 2.78, it is symmetric IUGR.
3. The symmetric IUGR occurs if the insult occurs in very early gestations, such as intrauterine infections (TORCH), trisomy and other genetic disorders

ADOPTED BABY

A 3-day-old adopted male neonate was brought to the OPD in neonatal department for routine examination. The baby was adopted legally from a government facility. The neonate was weighing 2.8 kg and physical features were suggestive of term gestation. Vital were within normal limits.

Questions

1. Enumerate your priorities during examination.
2. Name 2 tests for structural and nonstructural defects as part of screening examination?
3. Describe your drug advice to parents if maternal HIV status is not known.

Answers

1. As the neonate is otherwise is stable and no acute problems, the focus should be on issues which can effect long-term outcome.
   - Malformations
   - Any signs of infection
   - Any signs of trauma or fractures.
2. The investigations should focus on the above conditions:
   - ECHO, USG brain for structural defects, and hearing test and metabolic screen for nonstructural defect.
   - To screen for retrovirus and hepatitis-B
3. Administer nevirapine prophylaxis, it parents HIV status is not known.

GASTROESOPHAGEAL REFLUX

Case 1

A term male infant is brought to your OPD on day 14 of life weighing 3.9 kg with complaints of frequent regurgitation of feeds and abdominal fullness. Mother feeds the infant regularly every 2 hours. At birth, infant had a weight of 3.1 kg, no significant antenatal or immediate perinatal events and was discharged on day 3.

Questions

1. What could be the most probable diagnosis?
2. What relevant clinical evaluation you will do to confirm this diagnosis?
3. How will you manage this baby?

Answers

1. Most probable cause is gastroesophageal reflux (GER) due to overfeeding since there is excess weight gain in the presence of feed regurgitation.
2. Clinical evaluation
   - History—detailed feeding history including timing of feeds, pattern, feeding position, proper burping. Also exclude other causes—any forceful vomiting, sleep disturbance, irritability and stool pattern.
   - Examination—general assessment of well being, examination for tense abdomen, visible mass or peristalsis, presence of bowel sounds to exclude other serious pathology.
3. GER is a benign condition seen in newborn period, peaks by 3 months and spontaneously resolves by 6 months to 1 year. The treatment involves:
   - Correction of feeding methods
   - Switch to demand feeding
   - Proper burping
   - Prone and lateral positioning and reassurance will usually be adequate
   - Pharmacologic measures like prokinetics or proton pump inhibitors are not indicated.

Case 2

An infant has spells of opisthotonic posturing, stiffening, with staring looks and jerking of extremities. These episodes are more frequent mostly ½ hour after feeds.

Questions

1. What is the name of this clinical phenomenon?
2. What are the components of this phenomenon?
3. Why H_2 blockers are not indicated in such infants more so if the infant is VLBW?

Answers

1. Sandifer syndrome with gastroesophagial reflux
2. Components of Sandifer syndrome include:
   - Spasmodic torsional dystonia with arching of the back and rigid opisthotonic posturing mainly involving the neck, back, and upper extremities
   - Symptomatic gastroesophageal reflux
   - Esophagitis, and
   - Hiatal hernia
3. Use of H_2 Blockers is associated with necrotizing enterocolitis in very low birth weight infants.

Case 3

A 54 days old infant born at 30 weeks of gestation is admitted with complaints of cough, breathing difficulty with history of on and off spitting after feeds, not gaining weight adequately with frequent arching of limbs. Infant was on oxygen support till 32 days of life. The treating physician made a diagnosis of aspiration pneumonia on admission.

Questions

1. What is the probable disease causing aspiration? Justify.
2. What are the nonpharmacological interventions, in the management of this infant?
3. Is there any specific treatment for this condition?

Answers

1. Aspiration pneumonia following gastroesophageal reflux disease (GERD) is the probable diagnosis. GERD is usually associated with micro/macro-aspirations in infants is associated with BPD. GERD presents infants as spitting of feeds, not gaining weight adequately with arching of limbs.
2. Nonpharmacological interventions include:
   - Positioning in left lateral or prone position
   - Thickening of feeds
   - Avoid overfeeding
   - Giving small frequent feeds
   - Nasogastric feeding may aggravate GERD.

3. Specific treatment: No currently available pharmacological methods is proven safe and effective in infants in the management of GERD. Surgical fundoplication is tried rarely in severe cases.

Case 4

A 4-week-old-male infant possets after feeds especially when he lies on his back. The infant is thriving well and you suspect GER.

Questions

1. What are the four functional elements of lower esophageal sphincter?
2. What is the difference between posseting, regurgitation, and rumination?
3. What is the most appropriate action in GER (choose one only)?
4.
   - Barium swallow
   - Trial of gaviscon
   - Reassure parents
   - PH study
   - Trial of domperidon
5. What are the effects of orogastric tube placement and caffeine therapy in GER?
6. Proton-pump inhibitors are not usually indicated in GER. When is their use justified?

Answers

1. The functional elements of lower esophageal sphincter include crus muscle, intrinsic tone of the distal esophagus, intra-abdominal esophageal length and the cardiac angle (angle of His).
2. Posseting is nonforceful return of milk seen in all babies. Regurgitation is similar but involves larger volumes and may lead to GERD. Rumination is a chronic motility disorder characterized by effortless return of complete feeds due to involuntary contraction of muscles around the abdomen.
3. Reassure parents.
4. They may aggravate GER.
5. Clear evidence of acid related disease when proven by diagnostic studies, is the only indication for proton pump inhibitors in GER.

Case 5

A mother comes to your OPD with her 1 month old infant with complaints of persistent crying, irritability, back arching, and feeding and frequent awakening. Clinical evaluation was essentially normal.

Questions

1. What is the most probable diagnosis?
2. What are the two common factors that contribute to this condition? Why?
3. If left unattended, what are the likely complications?
4. What maternal nutrition intervention has been found to be effective in the management of some of these babies?

Answers

1. GERD
2. Supine posture (leading to immersion of GE junction) and relatively large volume feeding are the two common factors that contribute to GERD.
3. Likely complications of GER include failure to thrive, aspiration pneumonia, obstructive apnea and laryngospasm.
4. Trial removal of cow's milk and egg from the maternal diet has been found to be effective in the management of some of these babies.

THYROID DISORDERS IN THE NEWBORN

Case 1

Day 8-old-male baby (Fig. 20) presented with poor feeding, lethargy, excessive sleepiness and mild indirect hyperbillirubinemia. On examination, he had wide open fontaneles, umbilical hernia. Thyroid function test (TFT) revealed total T4: 3.2 mg/dL, Total T3: 47 ng/dL and TSH: 60 mIU/L. [Reference range for TFT—Total T4: 6–15 mg/dL, total T3: 70–250 ng/dL and TSH: 0.6–6.0 mIU/L].

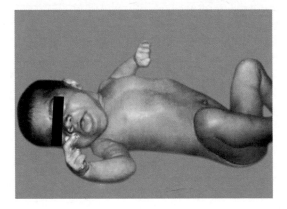

Fig. 20

Questions

1. What is your diagnosis?
b. What is the incidence of this disorder worldwide?
3. What are the two most common causes of this disorder?
4. At what age of intrauterine life, synthesis and secretion of TSH and T4 can be detected?
5. How treat to this disorder?

Answers

1. Congenital hypothyroidism
2. Incidence is 1 in 2000 to 4000 live birth worldwide
3. Thyroid dysgenesis (80%) and thyroid dyshormonogenesis (15%)
4. As early as 12 weeks of gestation, synthesis and secretion of T4 and TSH can be detected.

5. Treat with tablet L- thyroxine 10–15 µg/kg/day as a single dose in early morning and monitor thyroid function every two monthly during infancy.

Case 2

A boy born by normal delivery presented with jitteriness and convulsion on the fourth day after birth. His blood sugar was 30 mg/dL. On examination he had mild jaundice, cleft palate. His phallus was in-appropriately small for age. His free T4 is 0.07 ng/dL and TSH is 1.7 mIU/L.

Questions

1. What is your diagnosis?
2. What other investigations are adviced in this newborn?
3. What is the treatment for this patient?
4. Name any two genes associated with this condition?

Answers

1. Central hypothyroidism or secondary hypothyroidism.
2. Full hormonal profile including GH, LH, FSH, prolactin, and ACTH, Na, K and paired serum and urine osmolality.
3. In case of associated panhypopitutarism with ACTH deficiency, replace with hydrocortisone followed by thyroid replacement (to prevent addisonian crisis) till free T4 normalizes. Rest of the hormones can be replaced later
4. PIT-1, PROP-1.

Case 3

A term healthy newborn is subjected to thyroid newborn screening. On day 3 thyroid screening revealed Total T4: 2.8 mg/dL, total T3: 78 ng/dL and TSH: 3.3 mIU/L. Free thyroid hormones done on day 7 showed Free T3: 550 pg/dL, Free T4: 2.1 ng/dL, TSH: 3.1 mIU/L. [Reference range for TFT—Total T4: 6–15 mg/dL, total T3: 70–250 ng/dL and TSH: 0.6–6.0 mIU/L, Free T3: 170–760 pg/dL, Free T4: 1–2.6 ng/dL].

Questions

1. What is your diagnosis?
2. What is the inheritance of this disorder?
3. How will you treat this disorder?
4. How will confirm the diagnosis?

Answers

1. Thyroxine binding globulin (TBG) deficiency
2. X-linked dominant
3. No needs to treat this condition only reassure
4. Low values of serum TBG confirms the diagnosis.

Case 4

A term newborn with neonatal complications of birth asphyxia, gram- negative sepsis (requiring broad spectrum antibiotics), persistent ventilatory requirements and hypotonia is evaluated for possible hypothyroid status on day 23 of life. His Total T4: 7 mg/dL total T3: 34 ng/dL and TSH: 3.3 mIU/L. His Free T3: 90 pg/dL and Free T4: 1.5 ng/dL [Reference range for TFT—Total T4: 6–15 mg/dL, total T3: 70–250 ng/dL and TSH: 0.6–6.0 mIU/L, Free T3: 170–760 pg/dL Free T4: 1–2.6 ng/dL].

Questions

1. What is your diagnosis?
2. How will you treat this condition?
3. Which is the enzyme responsible for synthesis of T3 from T4 in brain and pituitary?
4. At what age of intrauterine life descent of thyroid gland gets completed?

Answers

1. Sick euthyroid syndrome or Low T-3 syndrome
2. No need to treat this disorder as it represents the physiologic adaptation to reduce oxygen demand and BMR in presence of ongoing catabolic process
3. Type II 5' deiodinase
4. 8–10 weeks of gestation.

Case 5

Baby A is a preterm infant born at 32 weeks of gestation to mother with Graves' disease. The baby presents on day 14 of life with poor weight gain, excessive crying but increased feeding. On examination, he has microcephaly, lid retraction, heart rate of 168/min and ECG is suggestive of sinus tachycardia. Thyroid profile showed TSH: 0.001 mIU/L. His Free T3: 30 pg/dL and Free T4: 0.2 ng/dL [Reference range for TFT—TSH 0.6–6.0 mIU/L, Free T3: 170–760 pg/dL Free T4: 1–2.6 ng/dL].

Questions

1. What is your diagnosis?
2. Which antibodies are involved in its etiology and disease severity?
3. How will you treat the condition?
4. How long treatment needs to be continued?

Answers

1. Congenital hypethyroidism or neonatal Graves' disease
2. Thyroid receptor stimulating antibodies (TRSAb) are involved in causation of neonatal Graves' disease. However, disease severity and its course gets modified depending upon levels of thyrotropin receptor- blocking antibody (TRAb).

3. Tablet propranolol (1-2 mg/kg/day, orally in 3 divided doses) and methimazole or carbimazole (0.25–1.0 mg/kg/day given twice daily).
4. Neonatal Graves' remits spontaneously in 6–12 weeks. Antithyroid medications can be safely tapered and omitted.

Case 6

An apparently normal newborn is noted to a large thyroid enlargement (Fig. 21). Mother was on antithyroid medication throughout her pregnancy. Her thyroid functions were normal.

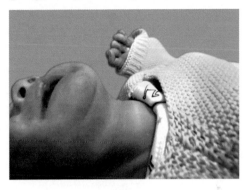

Fig. 21

Questions
1. What are different causes of neonatal goiter?
2. Will you treat this child with thyroid hormone replacement?
3. What is recommended dietary allowance of iodine in neonate and children?

Answers
1. Neonatal Graves' disease, iodine deficiency goitre, penderd syndrome, thyroid dyshormonogenesis, thyroid hormone resistance.
2. Depending upon his clinical status, If he is euthyroid then there is no need to treat; however, if there are compressive symptoms thyroid replacement to suppress goiter may be needed.
3. Recommended dietary allowance of iodine (RDA) 30 µg/kg/24 hr for infants and 90–120 µg/24 hr for children.

RETINOPATHY OF PREMATURITY SCREENING

Retinopathy of prematurity (ROP) is a leading cause of blindness. You are to lay down policy for ROP screening in your hospital.

Case 1

Questions
1. Which of the following babies would you exclude from screening program
    i. <32 weeks
    ii. Term hypoxic-ischemic encephalopathy (HIE) infants
    iii. 36 weeks with severe shock
    iv. 36 weeks with ventilation.

2. The best time to screen for infants >28 weeks gestation for ROP is.........
weeks of age.
3. Threshold ROP has a potential to cause blindness. It should be treated
within........days of detection.
4. Prethreshold ROP requires a return visit within ......days.
5. Planning is needed for lifetime follow-up of ROP. Name two visual
complications seen in childhood in ROP babies.

Answers

1. ii
2. 4
3. 2–3
4. 7
5. Squint, myopia, residual retinal scars (cicatrix), and retinal detachment.

Case 2

You are to review the treatment options for ROP.

Questions

1. .... is now the preferred mode of treatment for severe ROP.
2. The treatment of choice for cases of papillary dilation or vitreous hemorrhage
is ....
3. Name two treatments used to manage retinal detachment after ROP.

Answers

1. Laser.
2. Cryotherapy.
3. Scleral buckling and vitrectomy.

Case Scenario 1

Preterm infant with gestational age (GA) 30 weeks, birthweight 900 grams
admitted in neonatal intensive care unit (NICU). Baby is about to be discharged
at day 20 of life.

Questions

1. When would you like to do ROP screening for this baby?
2. What instructions would you like to give about feeding before for the screening?
3. Which eyedrops will you use to dilate the pupils?

Answers

1. Day 20: For babies with GA 30 weeks or less and or birthweight 1,000 grams
or less.
2. Instruct parents/nurse not to feed the child half an hour before and after
the examination.
3. Tropicamide 0.5% and phenylepherine 2.5%.

Case Scenario 2

For ROP screening refer Figure 22.

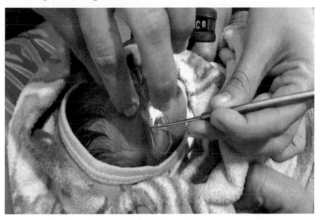

Fig. 22: ROP screening

Questions

1. When is the ideal period to screen a premature baby for ROP as per Indian criteria?
2. Name any two treatment options available.

Answers

1. Day 20: For babies with GA 30 weeks or less and or birthweight 1000 grams or less.

   Day 30: For babies with GA 34 weeks or less and or birthweight 1700 grams or less.
2. Laser, intravitreal anti-VEGF/Avastin (bevacizumab) injections and vitreoretinal surgery.

Case Scenario 3

For ROP screening procedures refer Figures 23 and 24.

Questions

1. Where should the screening be done?
2. When should the baby be fed before screening?
3. How do you dilate the pupils?
4. What are the instruments required for ROP screening?

Answers

1. Examination to be done in a clean temperature controlled environment. The procedure should be done under strict aseptic condition and with good monitoring facilities.

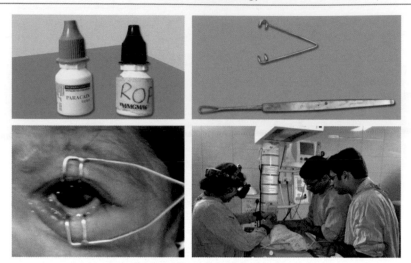

Fig. 23: ROP screening procedures

2. Baby should be fed one hour before examination to prevent vomiting and aspiration.
3. 2.5% phenylephrine and tropicamide 0.5% eye drops are instilled 2 times at 10 minutes interval about one hour before examination. Excess drops are wiped out to prevent systemic absorption.
4. Indirect ophthalmoscope, 20 D lens, pediatric wire speculum, wire-vectis (scleral indenter).

Precautions during the ROP procedure (Fig. 24)

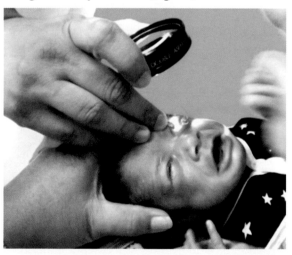

Fig. 24: ROP examination procedure

Questions
1. What are the complications during screening?
2. How to minimize stress-related complications during screening?
3. What local anesthesia drops to be used during examination?

Answers

1. Bradycardia, apnea, vomiting, aspiration
2. Routine use of topical anesthesia, nesting and sucrose administration
3. Topical paracaine (proparacaine) 0.5% eyedrops.

Preparation for Laser therapy (Fig. 25)

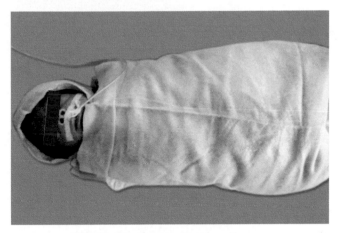

Fig. 25: Preparation for laser therapy

Questions

1. How many hours should the baby be fasting before laser?
2. What type of anesthesia is required?
3. Where should laser be done?
4. What steps should be taken to prevent complications?

Answers

1. Baby should be fasting 3 hours before procedure.
2. Topical anesthesia is used.
3. In NICU or in the operation theater
4. Vital sign monitor should be used. Emergency tray with intubation set should be kept handy.

Monitoring after Laser Treatment

Questions

1. When can oral feed be started after laser?
2. What are the complications during laser?
3. How long should the baby be monitored after laser?
4. What antibiotics should be given after laser?

Answers

1. Feeds can be started immediately if systemic condition is stable.
2. Apnea, bradycardia, hypoglycemia.
3. The baby should be monitored for 48–72 hours after the treatment.
4. Topical antibiotic drops should be instilled 6–8 hourly for 2–3 days.

Requirements for ROP Units

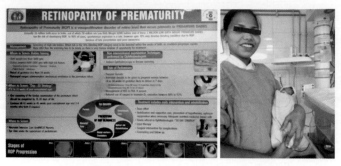

Fig. 26: ROP parent education leaflet

Questions

1. What forms should be available in NICU for ROP documentation?
2. What information should be given to the parents?
3. What is the role of nursing personnel in ROP screening and therapy?

Answers

1. Documentation forms with ROP chart based on international classification of retinopathy of prematurity (ICROP) with follow-up schedule, consent forms for screening and treatment.
2. Written and illustrated information for patients about ROP, the screening and follow-up process.
3. Primary counseling, preparation of baby and stabilizing baby during examination.

Case 3

Questions

Which of the following are not known to reduce the risk of vision treating ROP? (More than 1 is correct)
1. Prolonging pregnancy.
2. Intraventricular reduction.
3. Pneumothorax reduction.
4. Intervention bundle to reduce chronic lung disease.
5. Aggressive parenteral nutrition.
6. Oximeter alarm limits of 80–85%.
7. Avoiding oxygen saturations above 93%.
8. Transfusion thresholds.
9. Early surfactant therapy.
j. Head cooling.

Answers: e, i, j

Case 4

A 20-day baby is seen in OPD. You notice a bilateral opacity in the eye (Fig. 27). There is no corneal involvement, congestion, eye discharge or photophobia.

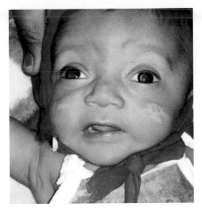

Fig. 27: Bilateral opacity in the eye

Questions

1. What is the most likely diagnosis?
2. When the condition is considered visually significant?
3. Which is the commonest in-utero infectious condition causing it?
4. Name the most common metabolic disorder associated with it?
5. What is the optimal time for intervention in unilateral and bilateral disorder?
6. What is the commonest etiology for unilateral affection?

Answers

1. Congenital cataract.
2. An opacity of the lens is considered visually significant when greater than 3 mm and centrally located.
3. Congential rubella.
4. Galactosemia.
5. Surgical intervention for congenital cataracts should occur within 6 weeks of birth for unilateral cataract and 10 weeks for bilateral cataracts.
6. Idiopathic.

Case 5

A 25-day baby has excessive watery discharge from both eyes. There appears to be photophobia (Fig. 28). There is no other anomaly. You find the following abnormality.

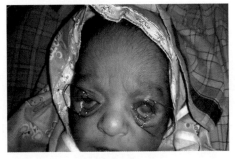

Fig. 28

Questions

1. What is the most likely diagnosis?
2. What is the underlying problem with this condition?
3. What test do you do to confirm your clinical suspicion?
4. What is the significance of the condition presenting at birth versus 3–12 months of age?

Answers

1. Congenital glaucoma.
2. Developmental abnormality affecting the trabecular meshwork.
3. Measure intraocular pressure.
4. Glaucoma that presents at birth is more difficult to treat, with at least half of the affected eyes becoming legally blind. Glaucoma that presents from 3–12 months of age has a favorable prognosis in 80–90% of cases.

STATISTICS

1. Standard guidelines for reporting of randomized controlled trials (RCT): choose one correct answer
   a. STARD
   b. CONSORT
   c. QUROM
   d. STROBE
   e. QUADAS

   Answer: b. CONSORT - Consolidated standards of reporting trials

2. Standard guidelines for reporting of COHORT study: choose one correct answer.
   a. STARD
   b. CONSORT
   c. QUROM
   d. STROBE
   e. QUADAS

   Answer: d. STROBE: Strengthening the reporting of observational studies in epidemiology

3. Standard guidelines for reporting of case control (TROHOC) study: choose one correct answer
   a. STARD
   b. CONSORT
   c. QUROM
   d. STROBE
   e. QUADAS

   Answer: d. STROBE: Strengthening the reporting of observational studies in epidemiology

4. Standard guidelines for reporting of diagnostic test: choose one correct answer.
   a. STARD
   b. CONSORT

c. QUROM
d. STROBE
e. QUADAS

Answer: a. STARD: Standards for reporting diagnostic accuracy studies

5. Standard guidelines for reporting of meta-analysis of randomized controlled trials: choose one correct answer
   a. CONSORT
   b. QUROM
   c. QUADAS
   d. PRISMA
   e. MOOSE

Answer: d. PRISMA: Preferred reporting items for systematic reviews and meta-analyses

6. Standard guidelines for reporting of meta-analysis of observational studies: choose one correct answer
   a. CONSORT
   b. QUROM
   c. QUADAS
   d. PRISMA
   e. MOOSE

Answer: e. MOOSE: Meta-analyses and systematic reviews of observational studies

7. From following Table from Trial of Indomethacin Prophylaxis (TIPP) study estimate

Outcome ⇒ Group ⇓	PDA	No PDA	Total
Indomethacin Group	142/ 601 (23.63%) (a)	459/ 601 (76.37%) (b)	601 (a+b)
Placebo Group	301/601 (50.08%) (c)	300/601 (49.92%) (d)	601 (c+d)

a. Relative risk (RR)
b. Odds ratio (OR)
c. Risk difference (RD)
d. Number needed to benefit (NNTB)
e. Relative risk reduction (RRR)

Answers
a. Relative risk (RR) = (a/a+b) / (c/c+d) = 0.24/0.50 = 0.48
b. Odds ratio (OR) = (a/b) / (c/d) = ad/bc = (142 × 300)/ (459 × 301) = 0.30
c. Risk difference (RD) = c/(c+d) – a/(a+b) = 0.50-0.24 = 0.26
d. Number needed to benefit (NNTB) = 1/RD = 1/0.26 = 3.84 = 4
e. Relative risk reduction (RRR) = 1-RR = 1-0.48 = 0.52

8. From following Table on PCR test in rapid diagnosis of sepsis calculate

Gold Standard ⇒ PCR Test⇓	Blood culture positive (Target disease present)	Blood culture negative (Target disease absent)	Total
PCR positive (Diagnostic Test Positive)	9 (True positive = a)	4 (False positive =b)	13 (a + b)
PCR negative (Diagnostic Test Negative)	0 (False negative = c)	87 (True negative = d)	87 (c+d)
Total	9 (a + c)	91 (b + d)	100 (a + b + c + d)

   a. Sensitivity
   b. Specificity
   c. Positive predictive value
   d. Negative predictive value
   Answers
   a. Sensitivity = a/a+c = 9/9 = 100%
   b. Specificity = d/(b+d) = 87/91 = 95.6%
   c. Positive predictive value = a/(a+b) = 9/13 = 69.2%
   d. Negative predictive value = d/(c+d) = 87/87 = 100%

9. Which is the ideal study design in the following situation: to estimate prevalence?
   a. Case control study
   b. Cohort study
   c. Randomized controlled trial
   d. Cross-sectional study

   Answer: d. Cross-sectional study

10. Which is the ideal study design in following situation—to determine natural history of disease?
    a. Case control study
    b. Cohort-study
    c. Randomized controlled trial
    d. Cross sectional study

    Answer: b. Cohort-study

11. Which is the ideal study design in following situation—in prevention or treatment of a disease?
    a. Case control study
    b. Cohort study
    c. Randomized controlled trial
    d. Cross-sectional study

    Answer: c. Randomized controlled trial

12. Which is the ideal study design in following situation—to study rare disease?
    a. Case control study
    b. Cohort study
    c. Randomized controlled trial
    d. Cross sectional study

    Answer: a. Case control study

13. Which is the ideal statistical test in following situation – comparing two treatment groups of different individuals with normally distributed numerical data?
    a. Chi Square test
    b. Paired or one sample t-test
    c. Unpaired or two sample t-test
    d. ANOVA
    e. Fisher exact test

    Answer: c. Unpaired or two-sample t-test

14. Which is the ideal statistical test in following situation–comparing two treatment groups of different individuals where numerical data is not normally distributed?
    a. Mann Whitney U test
    b. Paired or one sample t-test
    c. Unpaired or two sample t-test
    d. ANOVA
    e. Fisher exact test

    Answer: a. Mann Whitney U test

15. Which is the ideal statistical test in following situation—comparing two treatment groups of different individuals with nominal or categorical data?
    a. Paired or one sample t-test
    b. Unpaired or two sample t-test
    c. ANOVA
    d. Fisher exact test

    Answer: d. Fisher exact test

16. What is p value?
    a. Is the probability of finding the observed, or more extreme, results when the null hypothesis of a study question is true
    b. Is the probability of finding the observed, or more extreme, results when the null hypothesis of a study question is false
    c. Confidence interval
    d. Power of the study

    Answer: a. is the probability of finding the observed, or more extreme, results when the null hypothesis of a study question is true.

5

Drugs

ADENOSINE

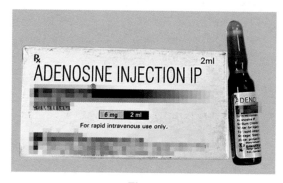

Fig. 1

Questions

1. What is the indication for this drug (Fig. 1)?
2. What is the serum half-life?
3. What is the dose?
4. How do you prepare solution for IV administration?
5. How do you give it?
6. What precautions will you take before administration?
7. What are the side effects?
8. How do you store this drug?

Answers

1. Treatment and diagnosis of tachyarrhythmia
2. Less than 10 seconds
3. About 50 μg/kg initial dose. Increase the dose by 50 μg/kg every 2 minutes. Maximum dose 250 μg/kg.
4. About 1 mL with 9 mL NS in 10 mL syringe (1 mL = 300 μg)
5. Give intravenous over 1–2 seconds followed by rapid flush of normal saline using 3 way stopcock.
6. Attach to continuous cardiorespiratory monitor. Arrange equipment for resuscitation and defibrillator

7. Arrhythmias, apnea, flushing, dyspnea, and irritability
8. At room temperature 2–8°C.

ADRENALINE

Questions

1. What is the dose of adrenaline in mg and in mL?
2. When to give adrenaline during newborn resuscitation?
3. Which is the preferable route of administration?
4. During newborn resuscitation, when is second dose of adrenaline considered?
5. What is the strength of adrenaline available in Indian market?

Answers

1. 0.01–0.03 mg/kg and 0.1–0.3 mL/kg of 1:10000 concentration
2. After 60 seconds of effective chest compressions with positive pressure ventilation, if heart rate is still less than 60
3. Intravenous
4. After 3–5 minutes of first dose, if heart rate is still less than 60
5. It is available as 1:1000 solution.

MAGNESIUM SULFATE

Questions

1. What are the indications of magnesium sulfate in newborn?
2. What do you monitor during magnesium sulfate treatment? -
3. What are the indications of magnesium sulfate during pregnancy?
4. What are the contraindications of magnesium sulfate?

Answers

1. The indications are:
   - Treatment of hypomagnesemia
   - Treatment of persistent newborn pulmonary hypertension (PPHN)
   - Treatment of torsades de pointes
2. Monitoring should include:
   - Heart rate and blood pressure
   - Serum electrolytes
   - Renal function
3. Indications during pregnancy:
   - In eclampsia
   - Neuroprotection in preterm delivery <32 weeks
4. The contraindications are:
   - Heart block or myocardial damage.

ERYTHROMYCIN

Questions

1. What are the indications of erythromycin in newborns?
2. What is the risk, if erythromycin is given in early newborn period?

3. What precautions should we take while giving erythromycin in newborns already on digoxin or aminophylline?
4. Why IV erythromycin is given slowly over 30–60 minutes?

Answers

1. The indications of erythromycin in newborn are:
   - Prophylaxis against ophthalmia neonatorum
   - Prophylaxis and treatment of pertussis
   - Treatment of feeding intolerance due to dysmotility
2. The risk of giving erythromycin is:
   - Increase in risk of hypertrophic pyloric stenosis by 10-fold
3. For those on digoxin and aminophylline:
   - Decrease in dose of digoxin or aminophylline as erythromycin may increase half-life of these drugs
4. The reason for slow infusion is:
   - Bradycardia and hypotension may occur rapid IV infusion.

LYOPHILIZED AMPHOTERICIN

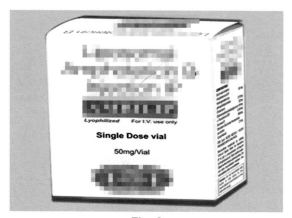

Lyophilized   For I.V. use only

Single Dose vial

50mg/Vial

Fig. 2

Questions

1. What is the dose for invasive candidiasis?
2. What is the mechanism of action?
3. Why does it cause less nephrotoxicity compared to conventional amphotericin?
4. What is the role of this drug in renal candidiasis?

Answers

1. 3–5 mg/kg daily intravenous for 3 weeks
2. Acts on ergosterol component of fungal cell wall causing cell membrane lysis
3. Binding to cholesterol in the kidney cells is reduced by the lipid formulation, hence reduced nephrotoxicity compared to conventional amphotericin
4. It should not be used in urinary candidiasis because of poor penetration of renal tubules.

AMPHOTERICIN

Questions

1. Lipid based and conventional formulations are interchangeable and have same dosing recommendations:
   - False
   - True
2. Lipid formulation have poorer penetration than conventional amphotericin into CNS, kidneys and eyes:
   - True
   - False
3. IV filters <1 micron should be used for amphotericin to prevent contamination:
   - True
   - False
4. Lipid form can be given in infusion with:
   - 5% dextrose
   - Normal saline
   - Half saline
   - Isolyte P solution
5. If baby develops hypersensitivity to amphotericin B deoxycholate, we can give lipid form:
   - True
   - False
6. What is dose of amphotericin B?
7. What is dose of liposomal amphotericin?
8. What 6 instructions you will give to nurse for amphotericin?

Answers

1. False
2. True
3. False
4. 5% dextrose
5. False
6. *Test dose*: 0.1 mg/kg IV, not to exceed 1 mg; administer over 20–60 minutes
   Initial dose: 0.25 mg/kg/dose IV/once daily
   Maintenance: Increase by 0.25 mg/day increments as tolerated to 1–1.5 mg/kg/day.
7. 3–5 mg/kg/dose/day for 3-week
8. Reconstitute 50 mg vial contents by adding 10 mL sterile water for injection (SWI) without bacteriostatic agent to obtain a 5 mg/mL solution-add SWI rapidly and shake immediately
   - Dilute further (usually to 0.1 mg/mL) with 500 mL D5W
   - Do not use, if precipitate or foreign matter is present
   - Store dry form at 36–46°F (2–8°C)
   - Protect from light
   - Use promptly after dilution
   - Infuse over 2–6 hours
   - May use an inline filter provided which has a pore diameter >1 micron
   - Use IV site in distal vein

CALCIUM GLUCONATE

Questions

1. How much elemental calcium does each mL of 10% calcium gluconate have?
2. What are the two important complications of IV calcium gluconate?
3. Name the drug given to pregnant mothers that may precipitate early onset-hypocalcemia in newborn.
4. Which other drug needs to be given, if hypocalcemic seizures are uncontrolled despite an adequate dose of IV calcium gluconate?

Answers

1. 9 mg/mL
2. Bradycardia and tissue necrosis on extravasation
3. Anticonvulsants
4. Magnesium sulfate

THIAMINE

Questions

1. What are the indications for use of thiamine in neonates?
2. What are the main clinical features of these conditions?

Answers

1. Maple syrup (MSUD), pyruvate metabolism disorders
2. Encephalopathy, metabolic acidosis

PYRIDOXINE

Questions

1. When is pyridoxine used in neonates?
2. When do you suspect this condition?
3. What is the dose of pyridoxine in such situations?

Answers

1. Suspected pyridoxine dependency seizures
2. Intractable seizures, reversal of EEG abnormalities following pyridoxine administration
3. 100 mg

ANTI-D

Questions

1. What are the indications for anti-D in a pregnant mother?
2. Do you give anti-D to the mother, if the DCT and ICT are negative in a Rh-negative mother?
3. How do assess Rh-isoimmunization noninvasively?

Answers

1. At 28 weeks and immediate postpartum (<72 hrs) in a Rh-negative pregnant mother who is still not isoimmunized
2. Yes
3. Fetal MCA Doppler plotted on the Marie curves.

DEXTROSE

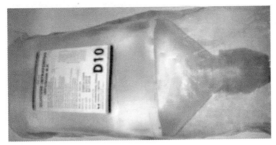

Fig. 3

Questions

1. Name two common indications for using this fluid in a neonate (Fig. 3).
2. What is the osmolarity of the fluid?
3. Name two common side effects of this fluid.
4. How many calories are provided by 1 mL of this solution?

Answers

1. It is used for fluid and calorie requirements in a neonate and for treating hypoglycemia
2. 505 mOsm/L
3. Thrombophlebitis and hyperglycemia
4. 0.4 cal/mL

DIAZOXIDE

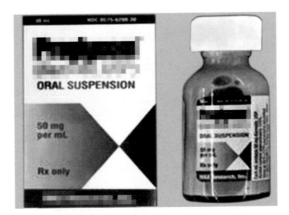

Fig. 4

A neonate has hypoglycemia with seizures at 6 hours of life. A bolus of 10% dextrose was given and glucose infusion rate (GIR) of 6 mg/kg/min was initiated. However, the subsequent hypoglycemic readings warranted an increase of GIR to the maximum of 12 mg/kg/day. Now, the baby is 12 days old and still is on GIR of 10 mg/kg/min. The neonatal team after some investigations decides to start on the above drug (Fig. 4).

Questions

1. What type of hypoglycemia best responds to the above drug?
2. What is the principal channel on which this drug acts, and how does it modulate this channel?
3. What is the dose of the above drug?
4. What is the serious side effect that needs the optimization of the fluid intake in the newborn?
5. What is the drug that is given along with this drug to overcome the above side effect?

Answers

1. Hyperinsulinemic hypoglycemia
2. Opening of the K (potassium) channels present on the surface of the beta cells
3. About 10–25 mg/kg/day in 3 divided doses
4. Fluid retention, hence fluid intake is restricted to 120 mL/kg/day
5. Chlorthiazide, this counteracts the fluid retention and suppresses the insulin secretion

MILRINONE

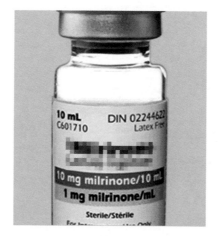

Fig. 5

A sick neonate, after a cardiac surgery, on moderate ventilator settings, is having shock. He is already on dopamine of 10 µg/ kg/min, but there is no significant improvement. The treating neonatologist plans to start the above drug (Fig. 5).

Questions

1. What is the mechanism of action of the above drug (mention the enzyme)?
2. What is the half-life of this drug?
3. What is the immediate and the most common side effect?
4. What is the primary route of excretion of the drug?
5. Name two indications for the use of the above drug.

Answers

1. Phosphodiesterase (PDE-3) inhibitor
2. Around four hours

3. Hypotension
4. Renal
5. (1) PPHN, (2) Low cardiac output states (especially after cardiac surgery), (3) Septic shock (cold).

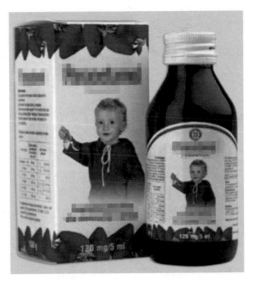

Fig. 6: Paracetamol syrup

A preterm infant with gestation of 28 weeks with respiratory distress syndrome (RDS) on mechanical ventilation is noted to have precordial activity, tachycardia and increasing oxygen requirement. A functional 2D-Echo done on this newborn confirmed hemodynamically significant patent ductus arteriosus (PDA). The urine output of this newborn in the past 12 hours was 0.9 mL/kg/ min. The neonatology team decides to start the above drug in this newborn (Fig. 6).

Questions

1. What segment of the prostaglandin synthetase does the above drug act on?
2. What is most common dosing schedule for this drug?
3. What is the chance of this baby having jaundice compared with Ibuprofen?
4. What are the current indications of using paracetamol in closure of PDA?
5. Efficacy of intravenous versus oral paracetamol.

Answers

1. Peroxidase
2. 15 mg/kg every 6 hours for 72 hours
3. Nil
4. When there is a contraindication of NSAID or failure with other drugs
5. Similar efficacy, however, some studies show IV is more efficacious than short oral regime.

FLUCONAZOLE

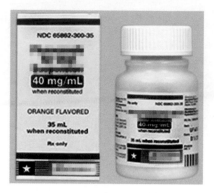

Fig. 7

Questions
1. What is the indication of prophylactic fluconazole?
2. What is the dose for prophylactic use?
3. What is the dose in treatment for candidiasis?
4. Is treatment dose dependent on gestation?
5. How is dose adjusted in renal impairment?
6. What causes gasping syndrome?
7. What is gasping syndrome?
8. What is concern, if administered with erythromycin?

Answers
1. Prophylactic fluconazole is indicated for very low birth weight (VLBW) infants in units with high incidence of invasive fungal infections (10%)
2. 6 mg/kg/dose twice weekly start at 48–72 hours of life and continue till 4–6 week/until no IV access required
3. 12 mg/kg/dose daily for 21 days for systemic candidIasis and 10–12 weeks for cryptococcal meningitis
4. No
5. If serum creatnine is more than 1.5, make prophylaxis once a week
6. Benzyl alcohol used in dosage form of fluconazole can cause gasping syndrome
7. Metabolic acidosis, CNS dysfunction such as convulsion, intraventricular hemorrhage and, hypotension
8. Prolonged QTc syndrome.

FOSPHENYTOIN

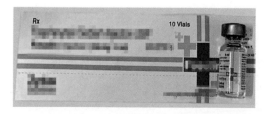

Fig. 8

Questions

1. What is the indication for this drug?
2. What is the loading dose and maintenance dose?
3. What is phenytoin equivalent of this drug?
4. What are the advantages this drug over phenytoin?
5. What are the significant side effects?

Answers

1. As an anticonvulsant for control of seizures in newborn
2. *Loading dose*: 15–20 mg/kg, *Maintenance dose*: 4–8 mg/kg once daily
3. 75 mg Fosphenytoin is equivalent to 50 mg phenytoin
4. The advantages over phenytoin are
   - More rapid infusion of intravenous loading dose (≥ 7 min)
   - Can be given intramuscular
   - Less irritant
   - Compatible with dextrose solutions
5. Irritant to skin, cardiac arrhythmias

INTRAVENOUS IMMUNOGLOBULIN (IVIG)

Questions

1. Name two prenatal fetal indications for its use.
2. What is the proposed mechanism of action?
3. What are the two indications for its use in managing immune-mediated hemolytic anemia?
4. Transfusion-related acute lung injury (TRALI) is a serious adverse reaction seen with IVIG. What is TRALI?
5. What is the role of IVIG in prevention of ABO incompatibility?

Answers

1. Alloimmune thrombocytopenia, severe erythroblastosis fetalis
2. IVIG binds the Fc receptor sites, thus competing with the anti-D sensitized neonatal erythrocytes and preventing further hemolysis
3. If the total serum bilirubin (TSB) is rising despite intensive phototherapy or B) the TSB level is within 2–3 mg/dL of the exchange level
4. Transfusion-related acute lung injury
5. No role

LINEZOLID

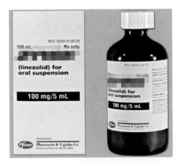

Fig. 9

Questions

1. Do you need to adjust the dose in renal impairment?
2. Linezolid is used in which infection?
3. What are the precautions required for IV infusion?
4. In which condition linezolid is contraindicated?
5. What one should monitor while using linezolid?
6. What is the major side effect in neonates and what is the cause?
7. For how long one can use linezolid after reconstitution?

Answers

1. Generally not required as excreted through liver
2. Vancomycin resistant enterococcal infection, and Methicillin-resistant *Staphylococcus aureus* (MRSA)
3. Precautions are:
   – Store at 25°C (77°F)
   – Protect from light
   – Keep infusion bags in overwrap until ready to use
   – Protect infusion bags from freezing
4. Phenylketonuria
5. Lactic acidosis, myelopsuppression, and hypoglycemia
6. Gasping syndrome. Caused by sodium benzoate added as preservative
7. 21 days.

LOW MOLECULAR WEIGHT HEPARIN

Questions

1. Name one use in neonates.
2. What is the route of administration?
3. What is recommended dose in newborn?
4. How to monitor for adverse effects for therapeutic dosing?
5. What is the antidote?
6. What are its advantages over unfractinated heparin?

Answers

1. Thrombotic conditions in newborn and proven cardioembolic arterial ischemic stroke, and in neonates with multiple cerebral emboli
2. Subcutaneous
3. 1.5 mg/kg/dose every 12 hourly
4. Anti Xa level of 0.5–1 unit/mL for therapeutic dosing and 0.35–0.7 unit/mL, 3–4 hours after subcutaneous dose
5. Protamine sulfate. If low molecular weight heparin (LMWH) was given within four hours, the maximum dose of protamine is 1 mg per 100 units LMWH, given by slow IV push. If LMWH was given more than four hours previously, then a lower dose of protamine should be used
6. Greater bioavailability when given by subcutaneous injection, longer duration of anticoagulant effect, clearance that is independent of dose (results in a more predictable response) and require minimal laboratory monitoring and dose adjustment.

NITRIC OXIDE

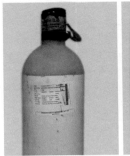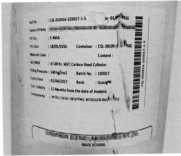

Fig. 10

Questions

1. What is the indication of this medication in newborn?
2. What are the indications for initiation?
3. What is the checklist before starting this medication?
4. What is the most important toxicity?
5. How do you monitor for toxicity?
6. How do you start?
7. What is positive response?
8. When to wean?

Answers

1. Used as pulmonary vasodilator in the treatment of pulmonary hypertension in term and late preterm infants (gestation >35 weeks)
2. PPHN, hypoxic respiratory failure
   - PaO_2 <100 mmHg on FiO_2 100%
   - O_2 saturations <92% on FiO_2 100%
   - Evidence of PPHN by echocardiogam and an FiO_2 requirement >60%
   - Oxygenation index (OI) ≥25
3. Checklist before initiation of inhaled nitric oxide
   - Lung volume optimized on chest X-ray
   - Surfactant is administered (if indicated)
   - Echogram to document PPHN and rule out other congenital heart defects
   - Hypotension corrected with vasoactive agents and volume as required
   - Baseline methemoglobin level
4. Methemoglobinemia
5. Level of methemoglobin after starting iNO should not be >5%
6. 20 ppm
7. The indicators of positive response are:
   - Increase in PaO_2 ≥20 mmHg or ≥ 20% from baseline
   - Increase in SpO_2 by ≥10%
   - Decrease in pulmonary artery pressure by ≥20% by echocardiogram
8. After 4 hours of stabilization and when the FiO_2 requirement is less than 60% to maintain SpO_2 >90%.

NORMAL SALINE

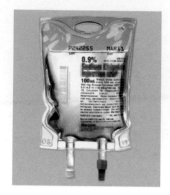

Fig. 11

Questions

1. What is the Na⁺ content in normal saline?
2. Use of normal saline during neonatal resuscitation is recommended. Name the indication, dose, duration and route of administration.
3. Name 4 common uses of normal saline in neonates.

Answers

1. Na – 154 mEq/L
2. *Indication*: When baby appears to be in shock and is not responding to resuscitation
   - *Dose*: 10 mL/kg
   - *Duration*: Over 5–10 minutes
   - *Route*: Umbilical vein
3. Common uses are:
   - Hypovolemic shock
   - Bolus of normal saline in all types of shock before initiation of ionotropes
   - Correction of dehydration
   - As fluid challenge in prerenal failure
   - In treatment of hyponatremia
   - As flush solution and dissolvent for many drugs.

DEXAMETHASONE

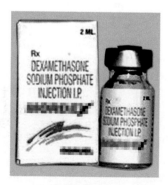

Fig. 12

Questions

1. Name two indications for use of dexamethasone in the antenatal period.
2. What is the dosing schedule of dexamethasone when used as antenatal steroids?
3. Name two most important neonatal morbidities that are significantly reduced with use of antenatal steroids.
4. What is strength of betamethasone vial available in India?
5. What are the indications for dexamethasone use in neonatal period?
6. Name three important short-term adverse effects of dexamethasone.
7. Name the most important long-term adverse effect of prolonged use of dexamethasone in preterm infant.

Answers

1. Indications for use:
   - Fetal maturation (Commonly known as antenatal steroids)
   - Treatment of fetus at risk of congenital adrenal hyperplasia (CAH)
2. Dosage for antenatal use:
   - Intramuscularly 6 mg, 12 hours apart for 4 doses
3. RDS and IVH
4. 4 mg/mL
5. *Postnatal use*:
   - In periextubation period
   - Treatment of postextubation laryngeal edema
   - Prevention and treatment of borderline personality disorder (BPD)
6. *Short-term adverse effects are:*
   - Gastrointestinal bleeding
   - Hyperglycemia
   - Hypertension
7. Poor neurodevelopment outcome.

BETAMETHASONE

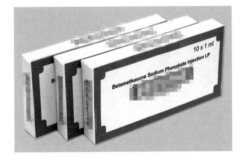

Fig. 13

Questions

1. What is the dosing schedule of betamethasone when used as antenatal steroids?
2. What strength of betamethasone ampoule is available in India?
3. Name three important short-term adverse effects of dexamethasone.

4. Name the most important long-term adverse effect of prolonged use of dexamethasone in preterm infant.

Answers

1. Intramuscularly 12 mg, 24 hours apart for 2 doses
2. 4 mg/mL
3. Short-term side effects:
   - Gastrointestinal bleeding
   - Hyperglycemia
   - Hypertension
4. Poor neurodevelopment outcome.

PROPRANOLOL

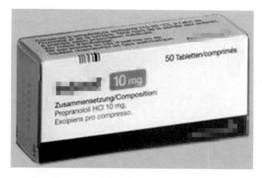

Fig. 14

Questions

1. Which type of drug is propranolol?
2. Which class of antiarrhythmic is propranolol according to Voughan William classification?
3. What are indications for use of propranolol in neonates?
4. What are the contraindications?
5. What is the dose?

Answers

1. Nonselective beta blocker
2. 1st generation class II
3. Indications for use in newborn are:
   - Supraventricular tachycardia (PSVT)
   - Tachyarrhythmias
   - Hypertension
   - Tetrology of Fallot's—cyanotic spells
   - Thyrotoxicosis
   - Large hemangioma
4. Hypotension, hypoglycemia, severe cardiac dysfunction
5. The doses are:
   - *Oral*:   0.5-1 mg/kg/dose
   - *Intravenous*:   0.01–0.02 mg/kg/dose

PHENOBARBITONE

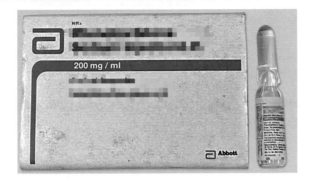

Fig. 15

Questions

1. What is the indication for this drug?
2. What is the loading dose and maintenance dose?
3. How do you prepare this drug for intravenous administration?
4. What precautions do you take while administration?
5. What is the elimination half-life?
6. What are the main side effects?

Answers

1. As an anticonvulsant for control of seizures in newborn
2. *Loading dose*: 20–40 mg/kg (20 mg/kg initial dose followed by 10 mg/kg in subsequent doses). *Maintenance dose*: 3–4 mg/kg once daily
3. Available in ampoules as 20 mg in 1 mL. Using 10 mL syringe, draw 9 mL water for injection and 1 mL injection phenobarbitone. Take the required amount, dilute and give over 20 minutes (not exceeding >1 mg/kg/min)
4. Be careful in babies with respiratory failure, preterm babies with gestation <28 weeks and in neonates with hepatic and renal impairment
5. 40 hours to 200 hours
6. Sedation, respiratory depression, and hypotension.

PROBIOTICS

Questions

1. Name one species of probiotics used for prevention of necrotizing enterocolitis in neonates.
2. What are the potential benefits of probiotic use in preterm neonates?
3. What may be the potential problems with routine use of probiotics?
4. What are the relative contraindications for use of probiotics?
5. When to start and stop?
6. Name any three mechanisms by which it may act and be beneficial.

Answers

1. *Bifidobacteria or Lactobacilli*
2. Reduced definite necrotizing enterocolitis (NEC), all-cause mortality and early time to reach full enteral feeds (~120–150 mL/kg/day)

3. The potential problems with probiotics are:
   - Sepsis due to strain of the probiotics
   - Lack of standardization of products and nonavailability of proven products in Indian market
   - Cross contamination within NICU with probiotic strains
   - Change in composition of breast milk when used with breast milk
   - Development of antibiotic resistance
4. The relative contraindications for use of probiotics are: Malfunctioning gut, sepsis, ileus, proven NEC
5. The ideal time to start is when the neonate is ready for enteral feeds, preferably within first 7 days of life and that to stop is at least until 35 weeks corrected age, or discharge
6. The proposed mechanisms of action are:
   - Increased barrier to migration bacteria and their products across the mucosa
   - Competitive exclusion of potential pathogens
   - Modification of host response to microbial products
   - Augmentation of IGA mucosal responses
   - Enhancement of enteral nutrition that inhibit the growth of pathogens, and upregulation of immune responses.

SILDENAFIL

Questions

1. Which group of drugs does it belong to and what is the mechanism of action?
2. What is the route, dose, frequency of administration of sildenafil in newborns?
3. Name one use in neonates other than PPHN.
4. Name a drug which may increase the concentration of sidenafil.
5. What monitoring is required when administering this drug?
6. What are the concerns for its use in extreme preterms?

Answers

1. Selective phosphodiesterase (PDE5) inhibitor. cGMP accumulation in pulmonary smooth muscle cells leads to pulmonary vascular relaxation. May potentiate action of iNO
2. *Oral*: 0.5–3 mg/kg/dose every 6–12 hours and
   Intravenous: Loading 0.4 mg/kg IV over 3 hours followed by continuous infusion @ 1.6 mg/kg/day (0.067 mg/kg/hour)
3. Severe Ebstein's anomaly
4. Fluconazole, erythromycin, and amlodipine
5. The monitoring includes blood pressure—watch for hypotension and oxygenation—watch for desaturation
6. Increased risk of retinopathy of prematurity (ROP) and platelet dysfunction.

VANCOMYCIN

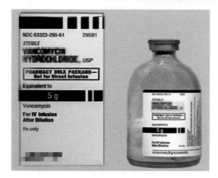

Fig. 16

Questions

1. If used with brufen or indomethacin should we:
   - Prolong the dose
   - Decrease the dose
   - Increase the dose
   - No need to do any change
2. Vancomycin levels should be:
   - Checked half an hour before giving the next dose
   - After 1–2 hour of giving the next dose
   - After 3 doses are given
   - All of the above
3. Why do we see trough and peak levels?
4. What is the ideal trough level for neonate with meningitis?
5. Dosing of vancomycin is dependent on?
6. How is dosing adjusted in renal impairment?
7. What are considerations for administration of vancomycin?
8. Red man syndrome (severe type) then what should be your response:
   - Stop vancomycin and give ranitine and diphendydramine
   - Never use it again
   - Slow the infusion over 90–120 minutes and increase the dilution volume
   - Slow the infusion over 90–120 minutes and increase the dilution volume and administer antihistamine before infusion
9. What are the routes of administration of vancomycin?
10. After reconstitution, we can store vancomycin for how long?

Answers

1. 1
2. 4
3. Trough level to see the adequate level for therapeutic effect and nephrotoxicity and peak for nephrotoxicity
4. 15–20 µg/mL
5. Postnatal age, weight and site of infection and renal status
6. Serum concentration monitoring with single dose administration in babies with urine output <1 mL/kg/hour or if serum creatinine increases from baseline (doubles)

7. Should be given in infusion over 2 hours and watch for Red man syndrome, which is hypotension, maculopapular rash
8. 1
9. Oral, IV, intraventricular
10. At 20–25°C after reconstitution with 5% dextrose or normal saline can store for 14 days.

ALPOSTIN

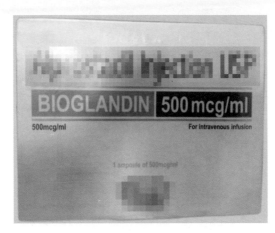

Fig. 17

Questions

1. What does this injection contain?
2. What is the indication for this medicine in newborn?
3. What is the dose?
4. What are the main adverse effects?
5. Name some conditions where alpostin usage may aggrevate clinical condition.

Answers

1. Alprostadil, i.e. prostaglandin E1
2. To keep the ductus arteriosus patent in neonates with congenital heart diseases such as isolated congenital heart defects that restrict pulmonary blood flow (pulmonary stenosis, pulmonary atresia), poor arterial-venous mixing (transposition of the great arteries), and defects that interfere with systemic circulation (interruption or coarctation of the aorta)
3. 0.05–0.1 µg/kg body weight/minute as continuous intravenous infusion
4. Apnea, hypotension, tachy/bradycardia, fever, and flushing
5. Obstructed total anomalous pulmonary venous connection (TAPVC), thermogravimetric analysis (TGA) with restrictive atrial septum.

6

Instrument

BILIRUBINOMETER

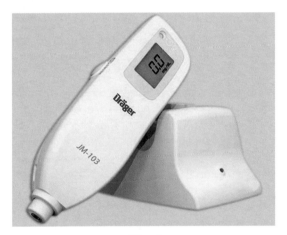

Fig. 1

Questions

1. What is the name of this instrument (Fig. 1)?
2. What are the best sites of measurement?
3. What is its principle ?
4. When is this machine most useful?
5. What are its disadvantages?

Answers

1. Transcutaneous bilirubinometer.
2. Forehead and upper part of sternum.
3. Measures bilirubin by spectrum of light reflected from the skin.
4. As a screening test and when the bilirubin is less than <13 mg/dL
5. High cost, not accurate at higher cut-offs, not accurate after starting phototherapy.

FiO₂ MONITOR

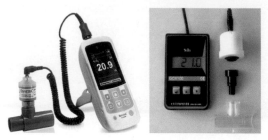

Fig. 2

Questions

1. Identify this instrument (Fig. 2) and its use.
2. What are the types of sensors used?
3. Where to place the probe when hood oxygen is being given for a baby?
4. Where to place the probe when baby is being mechanically ventilated?
5. What should be checked prior to its use?
6. What are the hazards of unmonitored oxygen therapy in the acute stage, short-term and long-term?

Answers

1. FiO₂ monitor (Fig. 2) or oxygen analyzer is used to monitor FiO₂ in certain high-flow oxygen delivery systems which do not have inbuilt analyzers like hoods, incubators and ventilators.
2. Electrochemical sensors: Polarographic (Clark cell) sensors and Galvanic (Fuel cell) sensors.
3. Close to the face at the bottom of the enclosure (Oxygen is heavier than nitrogen and it tends to settle down).
4. Before/upstream to active humidification system (condensation in sensors give erroneous readings).
5. Check if it is 21% in room air (if not, calibrate). Ideally also shows 100% with 100% oxygen.
6. Acute—failure to identify early worsening, short-term—free radical diseases of newborn (BPD, NEC, ROP); Long-term—associated complications of ROP, BPD (Visual deficit, motor deficit, behavioral issues, etc.)

FLUXMETER

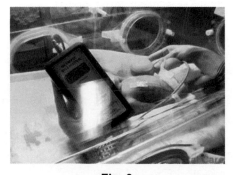

Fig. 3

Questions

1. Name the equipment shown in the photograph (Fig. 3).
2. When is this instrument used in the NICU?
3. What is the unit of measurement?
4. What is the definition of intensive phototherapy?

Answers

1. Radiometer/Fluxmeter/Irradiance meter.
2. To measure irradiance of a phototherapy unit.
3. $\mu W/cm^2/nm$.
4. Phototherapy delivered to the newborn at an irradiance of 30 $\mu W/cm^2/nm$.

NEONATAL INCUBATOR

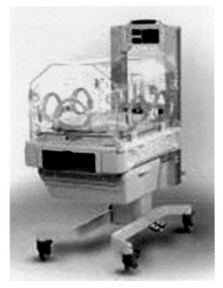

Fig. 4

Questions

1. What is the principle on which this machine (Fig. 4) works?
2. What are the definite indications?
3. What is the advantage over open care system?
4. When the baby can be weaned from incubator to open care system?
5. What are the disadvantages of this device?

Answers

1. Forced convection.
2. Gestational age <35 weeks and or birth weight <1800 grams.
3. Humidification, controlled oxygen and decreased radiant heat loss.
4. In skin mode, if heater output is <25% or in air mode at 30°C, baby maintains normal temperature for 24 hours.
5. Infection, high cost, and space occupying.

INFUSION PUMP

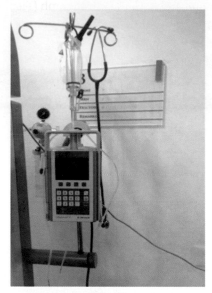

Fig. 5

Questions

1. Identify this instrument used in the newborn (Fig. 5).
2. What is the indication for use of this instrument?
3. What are the available types of this machine?
4. What is the mechanism of action?
5. What are the limitations of using this instrument?

Answers

1. Infusion pump
2. The indication for use of this machine in newborn is:
   - To infuse accurate and small amount of fluid or drug to the patients (babies)
3. Gravity-controlled pump and positive-displacement pumps
4. The mechanism of action includes:
   - The first type works on the basis of gravity and infusion rate depends on the pressure difference across the valve, i.e. height of fluid or venous pressure and a drop sensor is attached to the drip chamber to sense the drip rate.
   - The second type works with the help of a motor that helps to provide a positive-displacement of fluid, the positive-displacement mechanism is either peristaltic (linear or rotator) or piston.
5. The limitations of using this instrument include:
   - Occlusion alarm cannot detect infiltration/extravasation and so without proper line monitoring, infiltration injury may occur.
   - Biomedical back-up and technical knowledge required for smooth use.

MULTICHANNEL (MULTI-PARAMETER) MONITOR

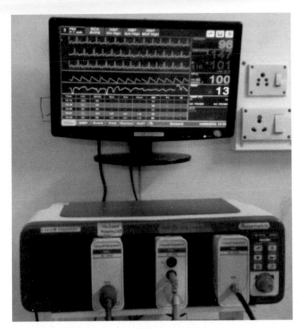

Fig. 6

Questions

1. What are the basic parameters that are measured by a vital parameter multichannel monitor?
2. What are the optional parameters that can be measured by these monitors?
3. What are the advantages of this type of monitor (Fig. 6) as compared to uni/biparameter monitors?
4. What are the disadvantages compared to uni/biparameter monitors?

Answers

1. HR, respiration rate, SpO_2, NIBP, and ECG
2. Temperature (skin and invasive), invasive BP, $EtCO_2$
3. The advantages of this monitor are:
   - Point-of-care monitoring of multiple vital parameters
   - Trends
   - Alarms
   - Long-distance connectivity for telemedicine
4. The disadvantages are:
   - Bulky
   - Expensive
   - All parameters may not be required for all patients
   - If one parameter is malfunctioning, entire machine has to be removed for repair

PHOTOTHERAPY UNIT

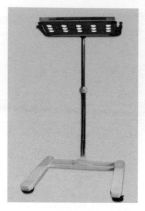

Fig. 7

Questions

1. Identify the instrument (Fig. 7) and the type.
2. What are the advantages of this unit over the conventional one?
3. What are the disadvantages of this unit over the conventional one?
4. Which instrument is used to measure the irradiance from this?
5. What is the minimum distance between the baby and the unit?

Answers

1. LED phototherapy unit.
2. Less heat generation and trans-epidermal water loss, non-fragile (no glass parts), low energy consumption, durable, no flickering (as it uses DC power supply) and hence no nausea or dizziness in healthcare professionals.
3. High cost, footprint area may be reduced by lowering the distance between baby and unit, possible increased DNA damage (in comparison with non LED units).
4. Fluxmeter.
5. 20 cm or closer but sufficient to observe the newborn.

PULSE OXIMETER

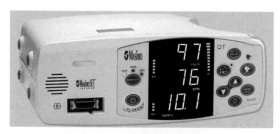

Fig. 8

Questions

1. How to judge the accuracy of saturation on the pulse oximeter?
2. What are the advantage of SET (signal extraction technology) over conventional technology?

3. At what SpO_2 range pulse oximeter is most reliable?
4. What is the law of pulse oximetry?
5. Which ambient light interferes with readings?
6. What is the limitation of this instrument?
7. What are the causes of preductal and postductal saturation difference in a newborn with cyanosis or low saturations or shock?

Answers

1. Heart rate correlates with baby's heart rate, pulse waveform is uniform.
2. Decreases low perfusion artefact and motion artefact
3. SpO_2 80–95%
4. Beer–Lambert law
5. Red spectrum, heating lamps, and phototherapy
6. Does not detect oxygen content or oxygen delivery. Unreliable with hypothermia, excessive movements, cyanide poisoning, methemoglobinemia, shock or low-flow state
7.
   - **Preductal SaO_2 = Postductal SaO_2**
     » Intrapulmonary shunt: PVR < SVR
     » Cyanotic congenital heart disease with L→R PDA: Ductal-dependent Qp: pulmonary atresia/stenosis, tricuspid atresia, and Ebstein's anomaly
     » PPHN: R→L shunt at PFO: PVR > SVR, ductus closed
   - **Preductal SaO_2 > postductal SaO_2**
     » PVR > SVR with R→L PDA: PPHN: MAS, RDS, CDH
     » Ductal-dependent Qs: HLHS, IAA, coarctation Anatomic PV disease: alveolar capillary dysplasia, pulmonary vein stenosis, TAPVR with obstruction
   - **Preductal SaO_2 ≤ postductal SaO_2**
     » TGV with pulmonary hypertension
     » TGV with coarctation of aorta

RADIANT WARMER

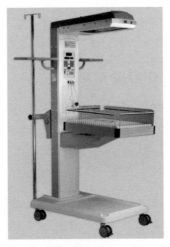

Fig. 9

Principle	Proportional heating device, provides heat by radiation
Role of parabolic reflector	Uniform heating across the bed of the baby
Role quartz or silicon rod	Quartz: slow heating and slow cooling silicon rod: rapid heating and cooling
Most important safety feature	When in servo mode, the temperature probe should always be on the baby
Role of rods under the heating element	Heat-resistant rods to prevent accidently burning of hands of caregivers
What are two places for fixation of temperature probe?	• Right upper abdomen above the liver when supine • On the flanks when in prone position
Indications for air mode or manual mode	• Prewarming • Resuscitation • Rapid warming of a severe hypothermic infant • During procedure
How to prevent evaporative heat loss?	• Use of a cling wrap • Avoid air currents in the NICU • Do not place warmers at entry and exit of NICU • Do not allow air currents from AC to fall on baby
What is the set skin temperature?	36 to 37°C temperature
When to remove from radiant warmer?	Heater output on skin mode <20%
Cleaning	• Dust with a clean cloth daily • After every use, when there is no baby, use 2% cidex, bacillocid or virkon.
When does a radiant warmer alarm?	• Probe failure • Baby temperature is greater than or less than 0.5°C from the set temperature • Power failure
Baby is having fever— Is this overheating or fever?	Warm peripheries: Overheating Cold peripheries: Fever

SELF-INFLATING BAG AND MASK

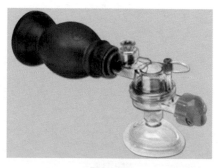

Fig. 10

Questions

1. Name the two safety features which must be present in every pressure-providing device.
2. What is the percentage of oxygen delivery, if the apparatus (Fig. 10) is held close to the patient's nose with oxygen reservoir and 100% oxygen?
3. Name two disadvantages of this apparatus as compared with flow-inflating bag.
4. What is the most reliable parameter for effective ventilation response?
5. How much should be the oxygen concentration at initiation during ventilation in < 35 weeks gestation?
6. What are your indications for stopping ventilation?
7. What do you do if the HR does not improve with ventilation?
8. When does first HR assessment take place after initiation of ventilation?

Answers

1. Pop-off valve and pressure gauge
2. 21% (it delivers oxygen only when the bag is squeezed)
3. Cannot be used to deliver oxygen, cannot deliver PEEP
4. Rise in heart rate
5. 21–30%
6. HR > 100/min with onset of regular spontaneous respiration.
7. Reassess ventilation – MRSOPA
8. When PPV begins, the assistant listens for increasing heart rate for the first 15 seconds of PPV

   Mask is tightly applied to the face.

   Re-position the head into the 'sniffing' orientation.

   Suction the nares and the pharynx.

   Open the mouth.

   Pressure of PPV can be increased to a more of 40 cm H_2O.

   Alternate airway, i.e. ET should be considered and planned for.

SYRINGE PUMP

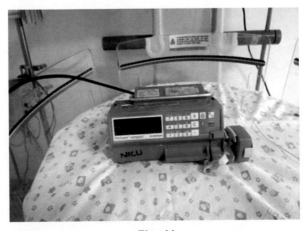

Fig. 11

Questions

1. Identify this commonly used instrument in the newborn (Fig. 11).
2. What are the main parts of this machine?
3. What is the mechanism of action?
4. What are the limitations of this machine?
5. What are the expected complications?

Answers

1. Syringe pump which is the most accurate type of infusion pump (type: positive-displacement pump)
2. Control panel, display panel, and driving unit
3. This pump works on a gear reduction mechanism with the help of a lead screw. It has a calculator mode, so that it can calculate the infusion rate as mL/min with the input of patient weight, drug concentration, and infusion rate as mg/kg/min.
4. The limitations are:
   - Cannot be used for large amount of fluid
   - Without technical expertise can cause error
5. The expected complications are:
   - Occlusion alarm cannot detect infiltration/extravasation
   - Without proper line monitoring, infiltration injury may occur

WEIGHING MACHINE

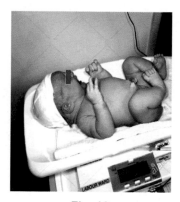

Fig. 12

Questions

1. What is the use of tare function on this machine (Fig. 12)?
2. What are types of weighing scales?
3. What are the weight range and accuracy of neonatal weighing machine?
4. How to clean weighing pan?
5. Which technique is used to avoid faulty weight by placement of baby?

Answers

1. To eliminate the weights of diaper and blanket on the baby
2. Spring balance and electronic weighing scales
3. 5-7 kg and +/– 1 gm (+/– 5 grams)
4. Disinfectants (Cidex or Savlon)
5. Load cell.

7

Imaging

INTERPRETATION OF CHEST X-RAY/ABDOMEN

Case 1

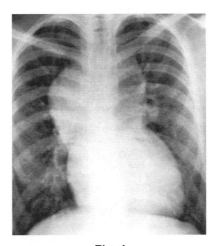

Fig. 1

Questions
1. What is diagnosis (Fig. 1)?
2. What is the sign?
3. What are the types?
4. On what feature does the clinical presentation of baby depend?

Answers
1. TAPVR due to an anomalous connection to left superior vena cava (SVC) shows the classic "Snowman" or "Figure of 8" pattern of enlarged supracardiac veins, left SVC, left innominate veins, and right SVC.
2. Snowman" or "Figure of 8".
3. Infracardiac, supracardiac, and coronary sinus or intracardiac variety.
4. Variable. Depends on the type of venous connections present and the *degree* of pulmonary venous obstruction.
   - Severe: cyanosis, respiratory distress, and tachypnea early after birth.
   - Unobstructed: poor feeding, failure to thrive, hypoxia, tachypnea.

Case 2

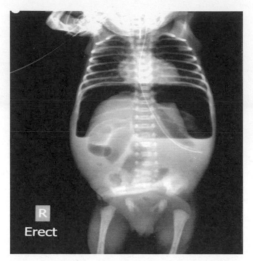

Erect

Fig. 2

A preterm of 27 weeks gestation, female baby, birth weight being 980 g with adequate antenatal steroid coverage, was born by emergency lower segment cesarean section (LSCS) for abruptio placentae, cried immediately after birth with no respiratory distress and oxygen requirement in immediate postnatal period. She developed sudden abdominal distension on day 4 of life (Fig. 2).

Questions

1. What are the differential diagnoses?
2. How do you distinguish between spontaneous intestinal perforation (SIP) and NEC?
3. What are the indications for surgery in NEC?

Answers

1. Differential diagnosis

Pneumoperitoneum-perforation of abdominal viscus
- Spontaneous intestinal perforation (SIP)
- Secondary to volvulus neonatorum, malrotation and meconium ileus
- Necrotizing enterocolitis (NEC).

2. Differences between SIP and NEC

Characteristics	SIP	NEC
Age at diagnosis	First week	2nd, 3rd week onwards
Clinical condition	More stable	critical
Pathology	Focal perforation without inflammatory component	Coagulation (hemorrhagic-ischemic necrosis of mucosa, submucosa and bacterial overgrowth

Contd...

Contd...

Mortality	Less	More
Area mostly involved	Terminal ileum or jejunum	Terminal ileum and ascending colon
Associated metabolic and hematological abnormality	none	Generally with new-onset hyponatremia, metabolic acidosis, thrombocytopenia

3. **Indications for surgery in NEC**
   - Intestinal perforation
   - Fixed a-dynamic loop of necrotic gut
   - Signs suggestive of necrotic gut-severe metabolic acidosis, persistent severe thrombocytopenia.

Case 3

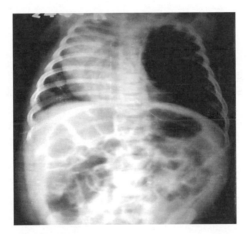

Fig. 3

A 24-day-old with birth weight of 2400 g, female newborn gets admitted with complaints of progressively increasing rapid breathing noticed by her mother since birth and occasional mild fever. Chest X-ray is given above (Fig. 3).

Questions

1. What is the diagnosis?
2. What is the most common site of involvement for this malformation?
3. What are the probable mechanisms of causation?
4. What is the best management option: surgical correction or serial observation?

Answers

1. CLE-Congenital lobar emphysema of left upper lobe
2. Left upper lobe
3. Bronchial obstruction by
   - Aberrant vessels
   - Congenital deficiency of bronchial cartilage

– Bronchial stenosis
– Redundant bronchial mucosal flaps.

4. If severe respiratory distress with cyanosis is present, excision of the involved lobe may be lifesaving.
   – Less than 2 months of age
      » Mild-to-moderate symptoms with no cyanosis on room air: serial observation.
      » Severe symptoms with CT chest showing severe herniation of lung; VQ scan: perfusion defect; bronchoscopy: abnormal : surgical excision.
   – More than 2 months of age
      » Mild-to-moderate symptoms with CT chest: mild or no herniation of lung; VQ scan: no perfusion defect; bronchoscopy: normal: conservative management with serial observation
      » Severe symptoms: surgical excision.

Case 4

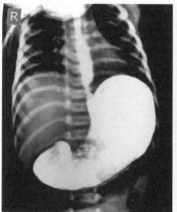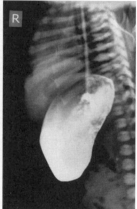

Fig. 4

A 28-day-old male, birth weight being 3000 g, with admission weight of 2400 g, full-term newborn presents with progressively worsening non-bilious vomiting, occurring immediately after feeding. Contrast study is shown above (Fig. 4).

Questions

1. Spot the diagnosis and differential diagnoses for the above contrast image.
2. Which electrolyte abnormalities are expected in this disorder?
3. Name the USG criteria used for the diagnosis.
4. Name the operative procedure which is most commonly performed?
5. A variable association was found with which drug when used in neonates?
6. Medical treatment with which drug is found useful in small group of patients?

Answers

1. Hypertrophic pyloric stenosis. Differentials are gastric outlet obstruction, hypertrophic pyloric stenosis, pyloric atresia and antral web.

2. Hypochloremic, hyponatremia, hypokalemia metabolic alkalosis.
3. Pyloric thickness >4 mm, overall pyloric length >14 mm.
4. Ramstedt procedure of pyloromyotomy.
5. Erythromycin.
6. Atropine.

Case 5

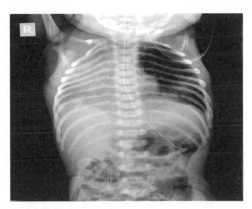

Fig. 5

A male newborn born at full-term with birth weight of 3100 g, came on day 10 of life with complaints of rapid breathing noted since birth by the mother. He was born to an unbooked mother and cried immediately after birth. On examination, breath sounds are not heard well on right side and heart sounds are better heard on right side. Chest X-ray is shown above (Fig. 5).

Questions

1. Describe (i) Findings and (ii) Differentials.
2. Name investigations for further characterization of this entity.
3. What are the complications expected at birth?
4. In cases of survival beyond neonatal period, what are the complications observed?

Answers

1. Homogeneous opacity in the right hemithorax, ribs are appearing crowded on right side, there is mediastinal shift with tracheal deviation towards right side.

   Differentials
   – Right side unilateral lung agenesis,
   – Collapse/consolidation of right lung because of total main bronchus occlusion from mucous or meconium plug, external compression by aberrant vessel, bronchial stenosis, kinking of right main bronchus caused by herniation into the mediastinum.
2. CT chest and CT angiogram, 2D echocardiogram and bronchoscopy.
3. Respiratory failure, pulmonary hypertension, congestive heart failure from associated congenital heart defects.
4. Recurrent pneumonia and reactive airway disease.

Case 6

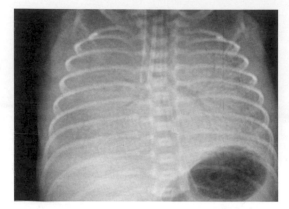

Fig. 6

Questions

1. What are the findings on this chest X-ray of preterm who started to have worsening respiratory distress soon after birth (Fig. 6)?
2. What is the diagnosis?
3. What are the specific interventions needed?

Answers

1. Findings
   - White out lungs (homogenous diffuse granularity)
   - Low volume lungs.
   - Air bronchogram extending peripherally
   - ET tube in right main bronchus.
2. Respiratory distress syndrome (RDS)
3. Increase positive end-expiratory pressure (PEEP), administer surfactant, and pull out ET tube.

Case 7

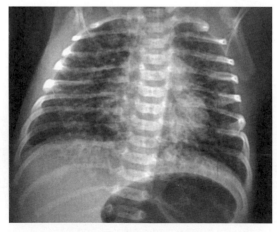

Fig. 7

Questions

1. What are the findings in this X-ray of newborn who presented with respiratory distress immediately after birth (Fig. 7)?
2. What is the diagnosis?
3. What are the two important complications associated with this disease?
4. What is role of antibiotics?

Answers

1. Diffuse, patchy infiltrates, areas of atelectasis and hyperinflation
2. Meconium aspiration syndrome.
3. Air leak, persistent pulmonary hypertension of the newborn (PPHN)
4. Antibiotics are used in view of the difficulty in differentiating it from pneumonia. But there is no consensus or recommendation.

Case 8

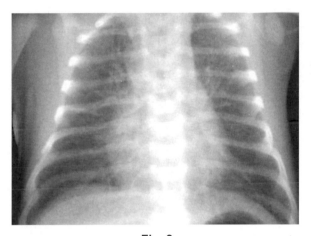

Fig. 8

Questions

1. What are the X-ray findings (Fig. 8)?
2. What is the diagnosis?
3. What are the risk factors for this condition?
4. How to confirm the diagnosis?
5. Which long-term pulmonary morbidity is linked to this disease?

Answers

1. X-ray findings
   - Streaky bilateral parahilar infiltrates
   - Prominent interlobar fissure
   - Hyperaeration
2. Transient tachypnea of the newborn (TTN) on the chest.
3. Delivery before 39 weeks, precipitous delivery (elective LSCS), maternal diabetes, fetal distress, and maternal sedation
4. Resolution of symptoms within 48–72 hours
5. Asthma.

Case 9

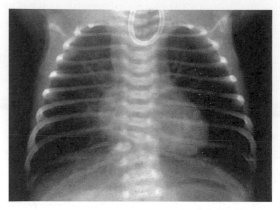

Fig. 9

Questions

1. What are the three X-ray findings (Fig. 9)?
2. What is the diagnosis?
3. Name a prenatal condition which is most commonly associated with this diagnosis?
4. What is the commonest type?
5. Complications of surgery.

Answers

a. Coiling of NG tube, D10 hemi-vertebra, presence of stomach gas bubble
b. Tracheoesophageal fistula with vertebral defects—probable VATER association
c. Antenatal polyhydramnios
d. Type C
e. Anastomotic leaks, strictures, gastroesophageal reflux (GER), dysmotility, and chest wall deformities.

Case 10

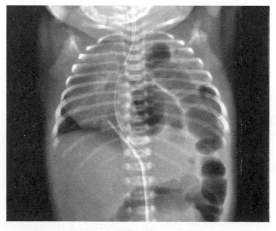

Fig. 10

Questions

1. What are the abnormal findings on this chest X-ray (Fig. 10)?
2. What is the diagnosis?
3. How would be the common clinical features of this condition?
4. What determines the survival?
5. What is PLUG?

Answers

1. Bowel loops in left hemithorax, mediastinal shift to right, and stomach (NG tube) in abdomen.
2. Left congenital diaphragmatic hernia.
3. Scaphoid abdomen, respiratory distress, mediastinal shift, and bowel sounds in the thorax.
4. Degree of pulmonary hypoplasia
5. PLUG is antenatal tracheal occlusion 'Plug the Lung Until it Grows'.

Case 11

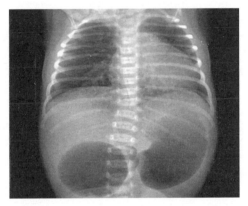

Fig. 11

Questions

1. What are the three abnormal findings seen on the X-ray of this newborn (Fig. 11)?
2. What is the diagnosis?
3. What is the commonest association of this condition?
4. What are the clinical manifestations of this abnormality?
5. How is it diagnosed antenatal?

Answers

1. X-ray findings
   - Double bubble sign (dilated stomach and proximal duodenum with absence of gas in the remaining bowel)
   - Abnormal D10 vertebra
   - 11 ribs on right side
2. Duodenal atresia with vertebral/rib defects
3. Down syndrome
4. Excessive of gastric aspirations at birth (>25 mL), nonbilious vomiting, epigastric fullness, and delayed passage of meconium.
5. Polyhydramnios and double bubble sign.

Case 12

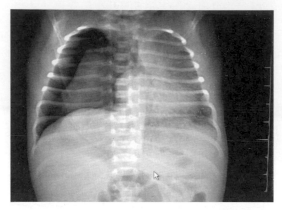

Fig. 12

Questions

1. What are the abnormal findings (Fig. 12)?
2. What is the diagnosis?
3. Excess of which ventilator parameter causes this complication?
4. What is the intervention needed?
5. What is the temporary measure done while making arrangements for the definitive intervention?

Answers

1. Collapsed lung with collection of air outside it in plural space
2. Right pneumothorax
3. PEEP
4. Intercostal drainage
5. Give 100% oxygen (to replace the nitrogen with oxygen in the collected space so that it gets easily absorbed).

Case 13

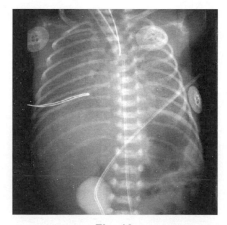

Fig. 13

Question

Comment on the tubes and lines on this chest X-ray (Fig. 13).

Answer

- Endotracheal tube is in satisfactory position
- The smaller tube next to ET is an orogastric tube and that is in the upper esophagus (too high)
- The umbilical arterial catheter (UAC) is also at high position at T4 (ideal is at T6 to T10).

Case 14

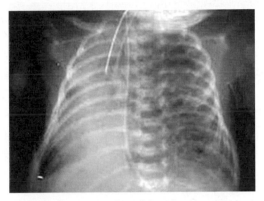

Fig. 14

Questions

1. What is the diagnosis (Fig. 14)?
2. What precaution should you take while resuscitating these infants?
3. Which is the most significant prenatal determinant of the survival outcome?

Answers

1. Left-sided congenital diaphragmatic hernia.
2. Direct endotracheal intubation without bag and mask ventilation and gastric deflation.
3. Lung head ratio.

Case 15

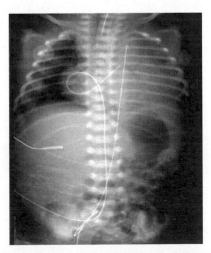

Fig. 15

Questions

1. What is abnormal in the X-ray (Fig. 15)?
2. What is the correct vertebral level of high and low positioned umbilical arterial line?
3. After inserting umbilical arterial line you notice blanching of right lower limb. What will you do next ?

Answers

1. High placement of umbilical lines with UV line looping inside heart and UA inserted too high (at T2 vertebra level).
2. High umbilical arterial line T6-T10, Low umbilical arterial line L3–L4
3. Warm the opposite limb. If no improvement in color of right lower limb remove arterial line.

Case 16

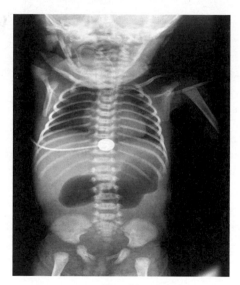

Fig. 16

Questions

1. What is the most likely diagnosis (Fig. 16)?
2. Give two differentials for this condition ?
3. What is the most common syndrome associated with this condition?

Answers

1. Duodenal atresia (double bubble sign).
2. Duodenal stenosis/duodenal web/annular pancreas/malrotation
3. Down syndrome.

Case 17

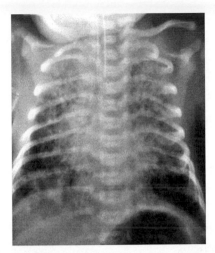

Fig. 17

Questions

1. Term neonate presenting with respiratory distress. What is the diagnosis (Fig. 17)?
2. What two complications do you expect while caring for this infant?
3. What is the latest recommendation in resuscitating nonvigorous and vigorous neonates born through meconium stained amniotic fluid?

Answers

1. Meconium aspiration syndrome.
2. Pneumothorax and pulmonary hypertension.
3. Avoid routine tracheal intubation and suctioning. Stabilization followed by intermittent positive pressure ventilation (IPPV) within 1 minute if required in both vigorous and nonvigorous newborns.

Case 18

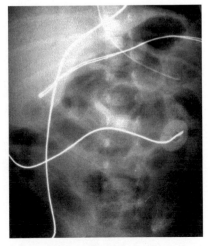

Fig. 18

Questions

1. What is the diagnosis (Fig. 18)?
2. What is the single most important risk factor for this condition?
3. How would you rule out free air in the abdominal cavity?

Answers

1. Necrotizing enterocolitis stage 2 (pneumatosis intestinalis)
2. Prematurity
3. Cross table lateral X-ray with horizontal beam/lateral decubitus X-ray or transillumination test.

Case 19

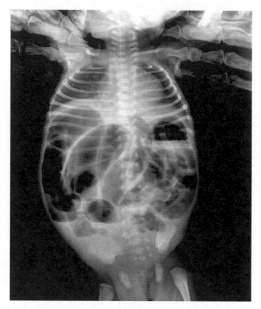

Fig. 19

Questions

1. What is the diagnosis (Fig. 19)?
2. Name two common signs with which neonates will present?
3. What is the most common differential based on the above X-ray?

Answers

1. Ileal atresia (dilated small bowel loops with air fluid levels)
2. Bilious vomiting/abdominal distension/failure to pass meconium
3. Hirschsprung disease.

Case 20

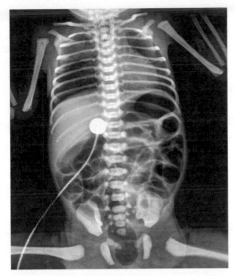

Fig. 20

Questions
1. What is the obvious finding in this X-ray (Fig. 20)?
2. What is the likely diagnosis?
3. Which is the commonest type?
4. How is esophageal atresia suspected antenatally?

Answers
1. Coiling of feeding tube in upper esophagus
2. Tracheoesophageal fistula
3. Blind upper end of the esophagus with distal end connecting with the airway.
4. Maternal polyhydramnios and absence of fetal stomach gas shadow.

Case 21

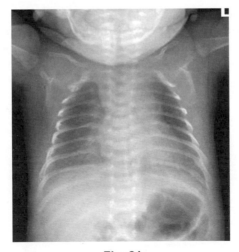

Fig. 21

Questions

1. What is obvious in this X-ray of a 26 weeker at 6 weeks of postnatal age (Fig. 21)?
2. Which is the most sensitive blood investigation to early diagnosis?
3. What is the main line of management?

Answers

1. Osteopenia of ribs, vertebrae, and humerus
2. Serum alkaline phosphatase
3. Oral phosphate supplementation.

Case 22

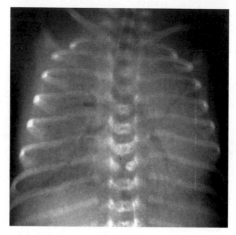

Fig. 22

Questions

1. What is the diagnosis (Fig. 22)?
2. What is the primary cause of this condiiton?
3. Which are the other differentials for this condition on the chest X-ray?
4. Name a cyanotic heart disease mimicking the radiographic picture?

Answers

1. Respiratory distress syndrome (RDS)
2. Surfactant deficiency
3. Group B *Streptococcus pneumonia*, pulmonary hemorrhage, pulmonary edema
4. Obstructed TAPVC.

Case 23

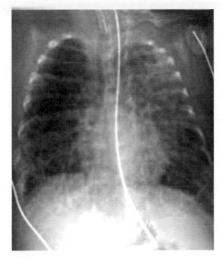

Fig. 23

Questions

1. This is a chest X-ray of newborn (Fig. 23) born at 26-week and at four weeks of postnatal age with ongoing ventilatory requirements. What is the diagnosis?
2. Which drug is prophylactically recommended in infants with this condition in first two years of life?
3. Which are the currently recommended pharmacological agents for prevention of bronchopulmonary dysplasia (BPD) in extremely low birth weight (ELBW) neonates?

Answers

1. Severe BPD with pulmonary interstitial emphysema
2. Palivizumab
3. Caffeine, high dose intramuscular vitamin A and aggressive enteral or parenteral nutrtion.

Case 24

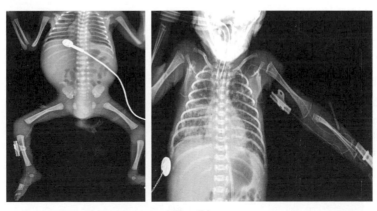

Fig. 24

Questions

1. Comment on the position of the peripherally inserted central catheter (PICC) line (Fig. 24).
2. What is the preferred position of PICC tip?
3. Which are the landmarks assessed to measure the proposed length of insertion?

Answers

1. LL (T 12 vertebral level), UL (T4 vertebral level)
2. UL PICC (superior vene cava–above T4) LL PICC (Inferior vena cava–below T9)
3. Upper extremity PICC (insertion site to 3rd intercostal space or sternal notch) and lower extremity PICC (insertion site to xiphoid process).

Case 25

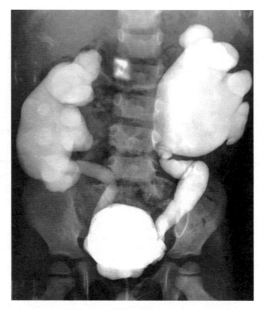

Fig. 25

Questions

1. What is the diagnosis (Fig. 25)?
2. What is the most common structural cause associated with this in neonates?
3. What is the treatment of choice?

Answers

1. Micturating cystourethrogram (MCUG) demonstrating bilateral grade V Vesicoureteric reflux
2. Posterior urethral valves
3. Urethroscopic fulguration of valves.

Case 26

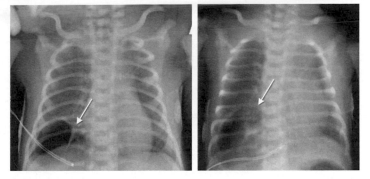

Fig. 26

Questions

1. What is the diagnosis (Fig. 26)?
2. What is the commonest presenting symptom in immediate neonatal period?
3. What are the factors affecting the prognosis?
4. What are the differentials for this condition on the chest X-ray?
5. How would you confirm the diagnosis?

Answers

1. CCAM (Congenital cystic adenomatoid malformation) or CPAM
2. Asymptomatic (type 1 CCAM—70% cases)
3. Cyst size <2 cm, associated anomalies like pulmonary hypoplasia, renal agenesis, cardiac malform (as in type 2 CCAM) are poor prognostic factors.
4. CDH, pneumatoceles, pulmonary sequestration
5. High-resolution computed tomography (HRCT) chest.

NEONATAL CRANIAL ULTRASOUND

Case 27

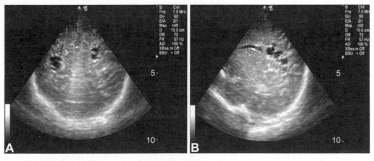

Fig. 27

Questions

1. Identify the view (Fig. 27).
2. Diagnose the condition.
3. Common causes of this condition.
4. Common complications of this neonatal condition.

Answers

1. Image A—coronal view, Image B—parasagittal view
2. Grade 3 cystic periventricular leukomalacia
3. Prematurity/VLBW/hypoxia/hypocarbia/PDA/Sepsis/chorioamnionitis
4. Diplegic cerebral palsy/intellectual impairment/visual disturbances.

Case 28

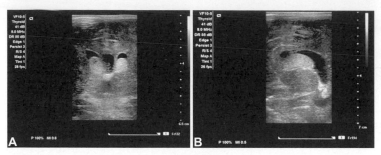

Fig. 28

Questions

1. Identify the view (Fig. 28).
2. What is the diagnosis?
3. Name the grading systems to classify this lesion.
4. Grade the image.
5. Best antenatal intervention to prevent this condition.

Answers

1. Image A—coronal view, Image B—parasagittal view
2. Image A—bilateral intraventricular hemorrhage, Image B—germinal matrix hemorrhage with intraventricular extension.
3. Papile and Volpe's grading systems
4. Grade 2
5. Antenatal steroids.

Case 29

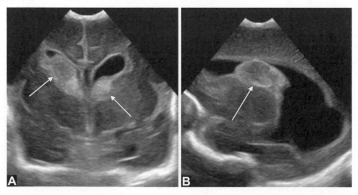

Fig. 29

Questions

1. Identify the views.

2. What is the diagnosis?
3. Grade intraventricular hemorrhages.
4. Best antenatal intervention to prevent this condition.

Answers

1. Image A—coronal view, Image B—parasagittal view
2. Intraventricular hemorrhage with ventriculomegaly
3. Image A—right side Grade III intraventricular hemorrhage/Image B—germinal matrix hemorrhage with ventriculomegaly.
4. Antenatal steroids.

Case 30

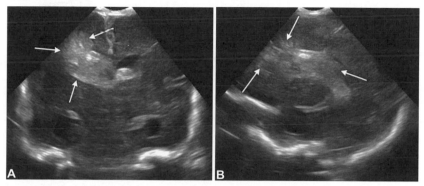

Fig. 30

Questions

1. Identify the view (Fig. 30).
2. What is the diagnosis on each of the image.
3. Best antenatal intervention to prevent this condition.

Answers

1. Image A—coronal view, Image B—parasagittal view
2. Image A—right-sided periventricular hemorrhagic infarction, left intraventricular hemorrhage. Image B—periventricular hemorrhagic infarction.
3. Antenatal steroids.

Case 31

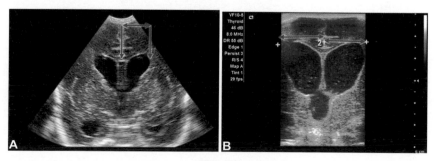

Fig. 31

Questions

1. Identify the view (Fig. 31).
2. What is the diagnosis?
3. Name the measurement index.
4. Drawback of this measurement.
5. What are the other measurements used for posthemorrhagic ventricular dilatation?

Answers

1. Coronal view
2. Ventriculomegaly—hydrocephalus
3. Levenes ventricular index
4. It may not go up during early hydrocephalus and the reference values for extreme preterm infants show variation because of less representation of this population in the reference curves.
5. Anterior horn width, thalamo-occipital distance, ventricular height, and frontal horn ratio.

Case 32

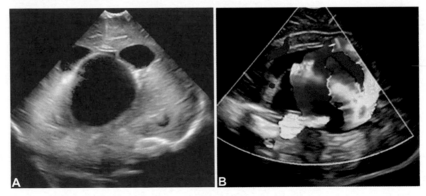

Fig. 32

Questions

1. Identify the view (Fig. 32).
2. What is the diagnosis?
3. What is the common presentation of this condition?

Answers

1. Image A—coronal view image, B—parasagittal view with color Doppler
2. AV malformation (Vein of Galen malformation)
3. High output cardiac failure (tachycardia, bounding pulses, bruit over the skull, cardiomegaly, and all four chambers dilated on the echocardiogram).

Case 33

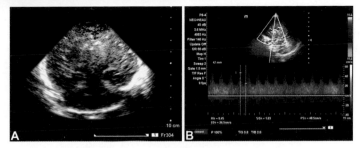

Fig. 33

Questions

1. Identify the view (Fig. 33).
2. How is resistive index calculated?
3. Normal RI value in term neonates?
4. What are the common causes of increased and decreased RI in neonate?

Answers

1. Image A—coronal view image, B—midline sagittal view with pulse wave doppler of the anterior cerebral artery
2. (Peak systolic volume-end diastolic volume)/peak systolic volume.
3. 0.65–0.9
4. Decreased RI—perinatal asphyxia, tachycardia, decreased cardiac output. Increased RI—PDA, hydrocephalous, pneumothorax, low arterial CO_2.

Case 34

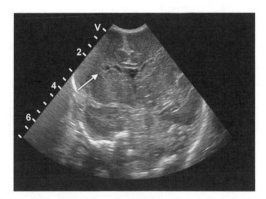

Fig. 34

Questions

1. Identify the view (Fig. 34).
2. Identify the arrowed structure. Give differential diagnosis and most likely diagnosis.
3. What is the clinical significance?

Answers

1. Coronal view
2. Cystic periventricular leukomalacia, connatal cyst, and subependymal cyst.
   - Most likely diagnosis is connatal cyst.

3. These cysts have been reported to resolve at follow-up studies without any clinical significance.

Case 35

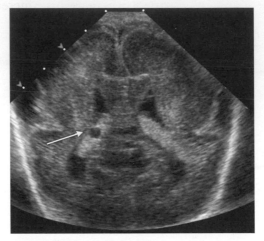

Fig. 35

Questions

1. Identify the view (Fig. 35).
2. Identify the arrowed structure.
3. What is the clinical significance of this isolated cyst?

Answers

1. Coronal view
2. Choroid plexus cyst
3. No clinical significance. It is a self-resolving lesion.

ECHOCARDIOGRAM

Case 36

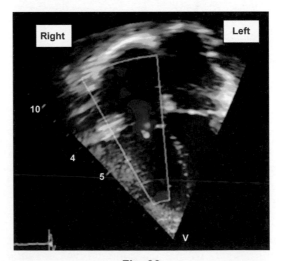

Fig. 36

Questions

1. What is the organ shown, which is the view (Fig. 36)?
2. What is the blue color jet signifies?
3. How does tricuspid jet quantifies pulmonary hypertension?
4. What are the common conditions where we have increase pulmonary pressures?
5. Which is the most common congenital heart disease to be ruled out if there is dilatation of RA/RV with high estimated right side pressures from TR jet?

Answers

1. 2D ECHO of heart, it is Apical 4 chamber view.
2. It is TR (Tricuspid valve regurgitation jet) and it signifies the quantification of pulmonary hypertension indirectly by estimating pressure gradient through tricuspid valve.
3. From the TR velocity the pressure gradient across the tricuspid valve is estimated using the formula $4V^2$

Method	Mild PAH	Moderate PAH	Severe PAH
TR jet estimated RV Pressures (mm of Hg)	30–50 mm of Hg	50–70 mm of Hg	>70 mm of Hg

4. Primary pulmonary hypertension (PPHN)
   Meconium aspiration syndrome (MAS)
   Severe respiratory distress syndrome (RDS)
   Severe birth asphyxia.
5. Total anomalous pulmonary venous return (TAPVR).

Case 37

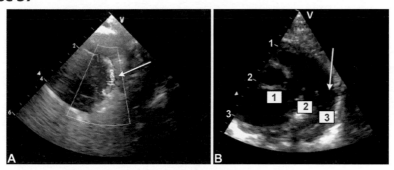

Fig. 37

Questions

1. What is being shown in color and 2D view marked by arrows (Fig. 37)?
2. What is the 2D view shown is commonly known as?
3. Name the structures 1, 2 and 3 in 2D view?
4. How you classify patent ductus arteriosus (PDA) on the basis of size?
5. What are the drugs used to treat hemodynamically significant PDA?
6. What is ductal steal and what does it signifies?

Answers

1. It is ductal view showing PDA (Patent ductus arteriosus)
2. In 2D view, it is called tripod sign
3.
   - Right pulmonary artery
   - Left pulmonary artery
   - PDA
4. Small <1.4, Moderate 1.4 to 3 mm and Large >3 mm
5. IV Indomethacin, IV and oral Ibuprofen, IV and oral paracetamol
6. Ductal steal is the reversal of the flow of blood in descending aorta during diastolic phase of the cardiac cycle, it is one of the component to define PDA as hemodynamically significant.

Case 38

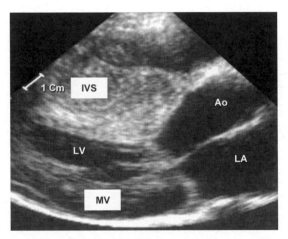

Fig. 38

Questions

1. Which is this view and what are the findings (Fig. 38)?
2. Newborn infant born at 40 weeks of gestation to a mother by emergency LSCS due fetal distress. The baby weighed 3.8 kg and cried immediately after birth. It presented with respiratory distress and weak peripheral pulses, X-ray chest is showing cardiomegaly, 2D ECHO is as shown, what is the condition?
3. If this infant have poor perfusion and low blood pressures with prolonged capillary refill time, how you will you manage?

Answers

1. Parasternal long axis view showing thickened interventricular septum and obstructing the left ventricular outflow.
2. It is hypertrophic obstructive cardiomyopathy (HOCM)
3. Frequent fluid boluses, vasopressin, and avoid using vasopressors such as dopamine, adrenaline or nor adrenaline. Propronolol is the drug of choice if there is no shock in the newborn.

MAGNETIC RESONANCE IMAGING

Case 39

Baby A, 28 week, 1.2 kg, male baby is born by normal vaginal delivery. Mother had severe PIH and baby needed resuscitation at birth. Apgar's at 1 and 5 minute were 3 and 7 respectively. During the NICU stay, baby had problems of RDS, *Klebsiella* sepsis and recurrent apneas. Neurosonogram on day 2 showed increased echogenicity around the ventricles. MRI at 10 weeks of age is in Figure 39.

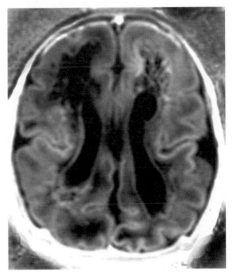

Fig. 39

Questions
1. What are the findings on the MRI?
2. What is the diagnosis?
3. What is the pathology in this condition?
4. What is the likely prognosis/Outcome of this baby?

Answers
1. T1 weighted image is showing bilateral hypointensive cystic lesions on the frontoparietal and similar lesions on the right parietooccipital area.
2. Periventricular leukomalacia.
3. Ischemia of the premature brain and white matter injury.
4. The baby is likely to evolve into spastic diplegic cerebral palsy.

Case 40

A full-term baby boy is born to a mother with gestational diabetes with a birth weight of 3.8 kg. Baby was admitted in the NICU for three days with one episode of hypoglycemia, and then discharged. At 10 days of life, this baby was admitted with seizures and MRI showed the following findings (Fig. 40).

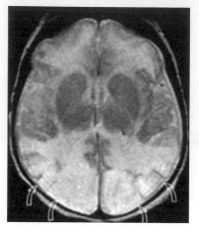

Fig. 40

Questions

1. Describe the findings
2. What is the cause of seizures in this baby?
3. How can you prevent this condition?
4. What is the expected long-term sequelae?

Answers

a. Abnormal hyperintensity in the parietal and occipital lobes on the T2 weighted image.
b. Hypoglycemic encephalopathy
c. Early detection of hypoglycemia in all high-risk babies (LGA, SGA, and late preterm), prompt, and aggressive treatment of hypoglycemia.
d. Spastic quadriparesis with cortical blindness.

Case 41

A term baby is admitted with seizures on day 1 of life and mother had no antenatal check-ups/monitoring. Initial blood investigations were all normal and the MRI scan showed the following (Fig. 41):

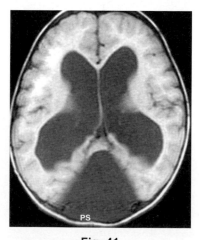

Fig. 41

Questions

1. What are the findings on the MRI scan and what is the diagnosis?
2. What are the three characteristic features of this condition?
3. What are the associated abnormalities?

Answers

1. Ventriculomegaly and cyst in the posterior fossa cyst (Dandy-Walker syndrome).
2. Agenesis or hypoplasia of the cerebellar vermis, cystic dilatation of the fourth ventricle, enlargement of the posterior fossa.
3. Hydrocephalus, atresia of foramen magendie.

Case 42

A term female child is born by normal vaginal delivery to a mother with A negative blood group. The baby was normal at birth, with Apgar's at 1 and 5 minute of 8 and 9 respectively. Baby developed jaundice on day 2 and progressed to have severe jaundice, seizures with irritability and hypertonia. Was treated with phototherapy and 2 exchange transfusions. MRI scan showed the following (Fig. 42):

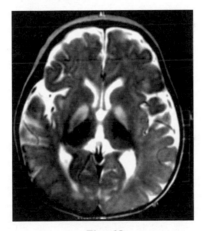

Fig. 42

Questions

1. Describe the findings on the MRI and what is the diagnosis?
2. What is the pathological reason for the above appearances?
3. How can you prevent this damage from occurring?

Answers

1. T2-weighted image showed hyperintensity at the basal ganglia region, diagnosis—Kernicterus (chronic bilirubin encephalopathy).
2. Bilirubin staining of the basal ganglia along with characteristic neuronal necrosis leads to the hyperintense appearance on the MRI.
3. Careful monitoring of babies for hyperbilirubinemia with risk factors
   - Intravenous immunoglobulin administration in the Rh sensitized neonate in the first few hours of life.
   - Early initiation and aggressive phototherapy
   - Prompt exchange transfusion.

Case 43

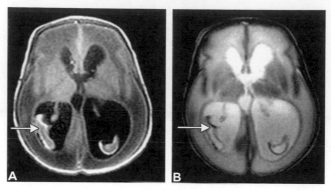

Fig. 43

Questions

1. What is the diagnosis (Fig. 43)?
2. Write the grading of this condition.
3. What are the complications that are expected with the above findings?

Answers

1. Bilateral Grade III intraventricular hemorrhage (ventriculomegaly and intraventricular bleed)
2. The grading of IVH includes:
   - Grade 1 – Germinal matrix hemorrhage
   - Grade II – Intraventricular bleed with no dilatation of the ventricles
   - Grade III – Intraventricular bleed with ventricular dilatation
   - Grade IV– Intraventricular bleed with parenchymal extension (venous infarction).
3. Posthemorrhagic hydrocephalus and adverse long-term neurodevelopmental outcomes.

Case 44

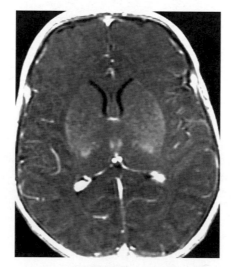

Fig. 44

Questions

1. Describe the findings in the above MRI image and what is the most probable diagnosis (Fig. 44)?
2. What is the most appropriate evidence-based treatment for this condition and when should it be started?
3. What are the criteria for initiating the above treatment?

Answers

1. Loss of differentiation of gyri and sulci and slit like ventricles–cerebral edema, hyperintensity if the caudothalamic region—ischemia, Most probable diagnosis—hypoxic ischemic encephalopathy
2. Therapeutic hypothermia (cooling) to be started within 6 hours after birth.
3. The criteria for therapeutic hypothermia in HIE are:
   - Evidence of hypoxia at birth—significant resuscitation for more than 10 minutes, Cord pH—<7.1, BE >–12.
   - Evidence of ischemia of multiorgan—deranged renal or liver function tests. (Not a criterion necessary for initiating TH, 1st and 3rd mandatory)
   - Evidence of moderate/severe encephalopathy using NICHD criteria—clinical seizures, or a-EEG evidence of encephalopathy or seizures.

Case 45

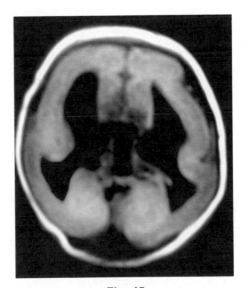

Fig. 45

A full-term 2.9 kg male newborn developed marked hypotonia and refractory seizures on day 1 after an uneventful normal delivery. He did not require resuscitation at birth. His weight, length and head circumference are between 50th to 90th percentiles. MRI brain is shown in Figure 45. EEG revealed bursts of sharp and slow-wave complexes, interspersed with periods of voltage depression.

Questions

1. Spot the diagnosis?

2. What are the conditions in which it is associated?
3. What is peak time period of gestational age for this kind of malformation of brain to occur?
4. What are the other disorders of neuronal migration?

Answers

1. Lissencephaly (i.e. "smooth brain")
2. Associations
   - Type I lissencephaly with chromosomal defects of 17p(LIS1), Xq(XLIS);
   - Fetal CMV infection
   - IEMs like pyruvate dehydrogenase deficiency, Zellweger syndrome, Glutaric aciduria.
3. The peak time period for neuronal migration disorders to occur is from 3rd to 5th month of gestation.
4. Other disorders of neuronal migration are:
   - Schizencephaly
   - Lissencephaly, Pachygyria;
   - Polymicrogyria
   - Heterotopias.
   - Focal cerebrocortical dysgenesis.

Case 46

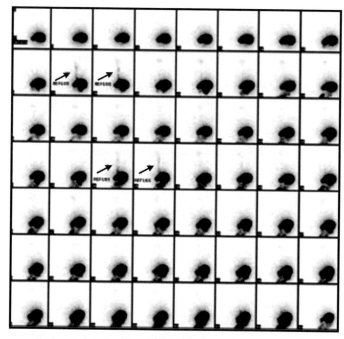

Fig. 46

Questions

1. What is this investigation and what does it show (Fig. 46)?
2. What is the condition called if the baby is irritable, has failure to thrive and symptomatic?
3. Mention at-least two complications of the above condition?

Answers

1. Gastric scinti-scan or milk scan, the scan shows that there is a significant gastroesophageal reflux
2. Gastroesophageal reflux disease (GERD)
3. Recurrent pneumonitis, Apparent life-threatening events, and failure to thrive.

Case 47

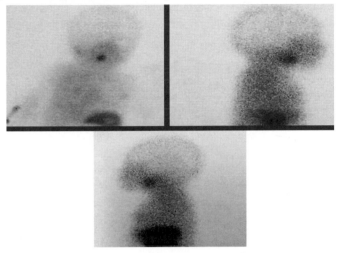

Fig. 47

A 2780 g female newborn was referred from a community hospital with history of not passage of meconium till day 5 of life. Her thyroid screening showed free T3: 1 pg/mL (0.91–3.92), free T4: 0.8 ng/dL (0.8–2), TSH (Ultrasensitive): 58 micro IU/mL (1.99–2.8). Thyroid USG neck was conspicuous for absence of thyroid gland in the neck. Thyroid scintiscanning with pertechnetate (^{99m}Tc) is shown above (Fig. 47).

Questions

1. Spot the diagnosis?
2. What is the dose of L-thyroxine used in newborns?
3. What are the precautions taken during supplementation of thyroid?

Answers

1. Lingual thyroid
2. 10–15 µg/kg/day
3. L-thyroxine tablets should be crushed and mixed in small amount of water or breast milk. Ferrous sulfate and soy-based formulas interfere with absorption, should be administered at least 2 hours apart from L-thyroxine dose.

Interpretation

ARTERIAL BLOOD GAS

Case 1

A day 1 preterm (31 weeks) newborn presented with respiratory distress and frequent apneic episodes. One dose of antenatal steroid was given 3 hours prior to delivery. There is history of preterm premature rupture of membrane (PPROM) for >24 hours

On examination: Heart rate (HR)—170/min, respiratory rate (RR)—70/min, capillary refill time (CRT)—4–5 sec

ABG revealed:

pH: 7.010

PCO_2: 24 mm of Hg

PO_2: 58 mm of Hg

HCO_3: 8 mmol/L

Base excess: -12.4

Questions

1. Interpret the arterial blood gas (ABG)?
2. What are the differentials for respiratory distress in this newborn?
3. What is the dose of antenatal steroid?

Answers

1. Partially compensated metabolic acidosis or uncompensated metabolic acidosis with normoxemia as pH is far away from normal
2. Respiratory distress syndrome (RDS)/Sepsis
3. Injection dexamethasone: 6 mg intramuscular 12 hourly × 4 doses or injection betamethasone 12 mg 24 hours apart for 2 doses.

Case 2

A day 2 term newborn presented with severe respiratory distress and is being ventilated. Emergency lower segment cesarean section (LSCS) was done for nonreactive cardiotocography (CTG). There is history of meconium-stained liquor.

On examination: HR—150/min, CRT—3 sec, Mean BP—48 mm of Hg

Ventilator settings: Mode: pressure control volume guarantee (PCVG), tidal volume—4 mL/kg, positive inspiratory pressure (PIP) max—24 cm, positive end-expiratory pressure (PEEP)—7 cm, FiO_2—0.75, RR—40/min

ABG revealed:

pH: 7.16

PCO_2: 57 mm of Hg

PO_2: 43 mm of Hg

HCO_3: 19 mMol/L

Base excess: -10.4

Questions

1. Interpret the ABG.
2. What is the provisional diagnosis?
3. Two drugs used for the condition.

Answers

1. Mixed respiratory and metabolic acidosis with hypoxemia
2. Meconium aspiration syndrome (MAS)/persistent pulmonary hypertension of the newborn (PPHN)
3. Sildenafil/inhaled nitric oxide (iNO)

Case 3

A term newborn is operated for congenital diaphragmatic hernia on day 4 of life. Currently baby is on the mechanical ventilation.

Ventilator settings: Mode: ACPC, PIP: 20, PEEP: 6, Fio2: 0.50, RR: 40/min

ABG revealed:

pH: 7.32

PCO_2: 53 mm of Hg

PO_2: 82 mm of Hg

HCO_3: 19 mmol/L

Base excess: -9.4

Questions

1. Interpret the ABG?
2. Name one important comorbidity?
3. Expand EXIT in the context?

Answers

1. Mixed respiratory and metabolic acidosis with normoxemia
2. Lung hypoplasia/pulmonary hypertension
3. Ex-utero intrapartum treatment.

Case 4

A term newborn presented on day 12 of life with signs of severe dehydration and ambiguous genitalia.

ABG revealed:

pH: 6.94

PCO_2: 26 mm of Hg

PO_2: 82 mm of Hg

HCO_3: 12 mmol/L

Base excess: -16.4

Lac: 7.3 mmol/L

Na^+ : 156 mEq/L

K^+ 5.5 mEq/L

Cl^-: 98 mEq/L

Questions

1. Interpret the ABG.
2. Write the formula for calculation of anion gap and calculate anion gap.
3. What is the screening method for this condition?

Answers

1. Uncompensated high anion gap acute metabolic acidosis
2. $([Na^+] + [K^+]) - ([Cl^-] + [HCO_3^-]$; Anion gap = 51.5 (High anion gap)
3. 17α-hydroxyprogesterone (17OHP) measured on filter paper blood spot (TMS) for congenital adrenal hyperplasia.

Case 5

A term newborn is being ventilated for PPHN.

Ventilator settings: Mode—synchronized intermittent mandatory ventilation with volume-guarantee (SIMV-VG), PIP—35 cm H_2O, PEEP—6 cm H_2O, FiO_2—0.90, RR—40/min, mean arterial pressure (MAP)—14 cm H_2O

ABG revealed

pH: 7.22

PCO_2: 50 mm of Hg

PO_2: 50 mm of Hg

HCO_3: 14 mmol/L

Na^+: 136 mEq/L

K^+ 4.0 mEq/L

Cl^-: 103 mEq/L

Questions

1. Interpret the ABG.
2. Calculate the oxygenation index (OI).
3. What is the indication of extracorporeal membrane oxygenation (ECMO) based on oxygen index (OI)?

Answers

1. Mixed metabolic with respiratory acidosis with hypoxemia.
2. 25.2 $\{$Oxygen Index (OI) = $\dfrac{FiO_2 \times MAP \times 100}{PaO_2}\}$
3. OI >40

Case 6

This is the blood gas of a newborn on mechanical ventilation.

ABG revealed:

pH: 7.30

PCO_2: 55 mm of Hg

PO_2: 75 mm of Hg

HCO_3: 30 mmol/L

Base excess: +6.5

Questions

1. Interpret the ABG.
2. What is the expected change in bicarbonate if PCO_2 rises by 10 mm of Hg (acute process)?
3. What is the expected change in bicarbonate if PCO_2 rises by 10 mm of Hg (chronic process)?

Answers

1. Primary respiratory acidosis with partial metabolic compensation
2. Acute: Bicarbonate increases by 1–3 for each 10 mm rise in PCO_2 in acute condition
3. Chronic: Bicarbonate increases by 3–5 for each 10 mm rise in PCO_2 in chronic condition.

Case 7

A preterm infant (32 weeks) on mechanical ventilation is noted to have pulmonary hemorrhage on day 3 of life.

Ventilator settings: Mode—SIMVVG, tidal volume—6mL, PIPmax—26 cm H_2O, PEEP—6 cm H_2O, FiO_2—0.70, RR—60/min

ABG parameters:

pH: 7.56

PCO_2: 23.7 mm of Hg

PO_2: 157 mm of Hg

HCO_3 (actual): 24 mmol/L

Questions

1. Interpret the ABG.
2. Calculate alveolar-arterial oxygen difference ($AaDO_2$).
3. What is the indication of ECMO based on $AaDO_2$ levels?

Answers

1. Mixed metabolic and respiratory acidosis with hyperoxemia
2. 384; Algorithm: $AaDO_2 = (713 \times FiO_2) - (pCO_2 / 0.8) - (paO_2)$*
3. $AaDO_2$ >620 for 12 hours on FiO_2 100%.

Case 8

23-day-old, female was rushed to the pediatric emergency following her mother's complaint that the baby is irritable, difficult to breastfeed and has diarrhea for the past 3 days. The baby's respiratory rate is increased and the fontanels are sunken.

The results from the ABG show:

pH—7.34, $PaCO_2$—27 mmHg and HCO_3—14 mMol/L, Na^+ = 166 mEq/L, K^+ = 4.0 mEq/L, Cl^- = 103 mEq/L

Questions

1. Interpret the ABG.
2. What are two important parameters of assessing hydration status of admitted newborns?
3. Calculate the anion gap. What is the minimum age when oral rehydration salt (ORS) can be given?

Answers

1. Metabolic acidosis with respiratory alkalosis
2. Weight and serum Na^+ level
3. Anion gap = 53 (High anion gap); no such age (even newborns can be given WHO approved low osmolar ORS).

Case 9

Consider the following two ABG cases:

Baby A	Baby B
pH: 7.48	pH: 7.32
PCO_2: 34 mm of Hg	PCO_2: 74 mm of Hg
PO_2: 85 mm of Hg	PO_2: 55 mm of Hg
SaO_2 95%	SaO_2: 85%
Hb = 7 g%	Hb = 15 g%

Questions

1. Write the formula for calculating arterial oxygen content.
2. Which of the above two babies is more hypoxic and why?
3. What is the normal value of arterial oxygen content?

Answers

1. $CaO_2 = 1.34 \times Hb\% \times SPO_2 + 0.003 \times PaO_2$
2. Baby A is more hypoxic as oxygen content of baby A is 8.9 mL O_2/dL and oxygen content of baby B is 17.1 mL O_2/dL
3. 16–22 mL O_2/dL.

Case 10

A preterm infant (gestation 29 weeks, birth weight 900 grams) is on mechanical ventilation for RDS not responding to INSURE (intubation, surfactant, extubation).

Ventilator settings: Mode—PCVG, tidal volume—8 mL, PIPmax—20 cm H_2O,
PEEP—6 H_2O, FiO_2—0.40, RR—60/min

ABG parameters:

pH: 7.14

PCO_2: 18.2 mm of Hg

PO_2: 67 mm of Hg

HCO_3: 15 mmol/L

Questions

1. Interpret the ABG.
2. What changes in ventilator parameters you suggest and why?
3. What are the risks with low PCO_2 in preterm babies?

Answers

1. Primary metabolic acidosis with superimposed respiratory alkalosis
2. Keeping tidal volume 4–6 mL/kg and decreasing respiratory rate to prevent CO_2 wash out
3. Periventricular leukomalacia.

CAPNOGRAPHY

Case 1

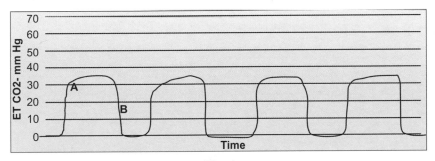

Fig. 1

Questions

1. Identify the graph and comment on its utility (Fig. 1).
2. Which phases of respiration are depicted in (A) and (B)?
3. What are the types of "sampling" used in $ETCO_2$ measurement?
4. Enumerate causes of low correlation of $ETCO_2$ values with $PaCO_2$?

Answers

1. It is capnograph. It is used for continuous monitoring of $PaCO_2$
2. A = Expiration, B = Inspiration
3. Mainstream and side-stream sampling
4. Reduced pulmonary blood flow, VQ mismatch, low tidal volumes and fast breath rates, low inspiratory time, and high dead space.

Case 2

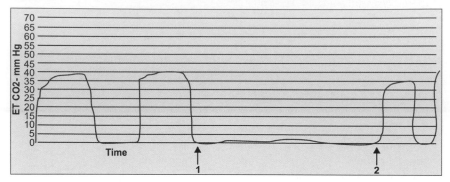

Fig. 2

Question

Name any two possible events that occurred between arrows 1 and 2 in a ventilated patient (Fig. 2).

Answers

1. Tube dislodgement (1) and subsequent reintubation into trachea (2)
2. Equipment failure and apnea (1) followed by resumption of respiration (2)
3. Cardiopulmonary arrest (1) followed by resumption of spontaneous circulation (2).

Case 3

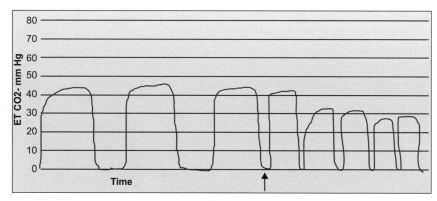

Fig. 3

Question

What could be the event at arrow and describe the change subsequently?

Answer

Onset of hyperventilation [spontaneous or intermittent positive pressure ventilation (IPPV)] followed by progressive fall in CO_2 measurements (reflective of hypocarbia).

C-REACTIVE PROTEIN

1. What is the most accurate method of estimation of C-reactive protein (CRP)?
2. What value of CRP (mg/L) is taken as threshold value?

3. What is the sensitivity, specificity and negative predictive value (NPV) of CRP in the diagnosis of sepsis?
4. What are the causes for false-positive and false-negative CRP?

Answers

1. The most accurate method is laser or rate nephelometry quantitative immunoassay
2. There is a strong statistical evidence to establish 1 mg/L as the appropriate threshold level, that is, the level at which the test has the maximum ability to identify infants with proven or probable sepsis. The serial CRP levels drawn 12–24 hours after the onset of signs and symptoms of infection are superior to a single level.
3. Serial measurements of CRP levels drawn every 24–48 hours after the onset of signs of infection have an increased:
   - Sensitivity between 78.9% and 98%
   - Specificity of 84–97%
   - A negative predictive value of 99% in detecting sepsis. A high negative predictive value indicates that CRP levels drawn between 24 hours and 48 hours can identify infants who are unlikely to be infected.
4. The causes for false-positive CRP are:
   - Maternal fever during labor
   - Prolonged rupture of membranes
   - Stressful delivery, fetal distress, or both
   - Perinatal asphyxia/shock
   - Meconium aspiration pneumonitis
   - Periventricular and intraventricular hemorrhage
   - Pneumothorax

   The causes of false-negative CRP are:
   - Preterm infants due to immature liver function
   - Overwhelming sepsis.

CARDIOTOCOGRAPHY

Case 1

A 25-year-old, gravida 2, para 1, live 1, mother presented with labor pains for 2 hours at 38 weeks of gestation. The cardiotocogram done at admission is shown below.

Questions

1. Interpret the findings (HR, variability, acceleration, and decelerations)
2. What is the expected outcome of this fetus?
3. What is the expected cord pH of this fetus?

Answers

a. This is a normal CTG
   - The heart rate is around 140 beats per min
   - Beat-to-beat variability is 5–15
   - Accelerations are present with fetal activity
   - Accelerations of 20 beats lasting for 15 seconds is seen

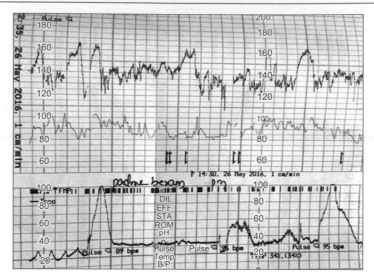

Fig. 4

b. This baby is likely to have a normal perinatal event. CTG has a high negative predictive value

c. The cord pH is expected to be above 7.25.

Case 2

A 20-year-old primigravida at 34 weeks of gestation presents with bleeding per vaginum. On examination of the abdomen uterus was active and corresponding to the period of gestation. Given here is the CTG (Fig. 5).

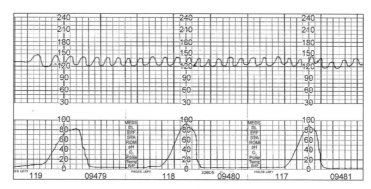

Fig. 5

Questions

1. What is the interpretation of the CTG?
2. What is the probable cause of this finding?
3. What is the preparation required for the management of newborn?

Answers

1. This is ominous CTG.
   - Baseline rate is 135 per min with a sinusoidal pattern showing 3–4 cycles per minutes
   - No accelerations or deceleration are seen
   - There is no beat-to-beat variability
2. Fetal anemia
3. O negative blood should be ready at delivery for resuscitation.

Case 3

A 30-year-old gravida 4, para 3, live 3 mother presented at 35 weeks of gestation with complaints of pain abdomen for 2 hours. Her antenatal scan revealed amniotic fluid index (AFI) of 2–3 cm, CTG done is as follows (Fig. 6):

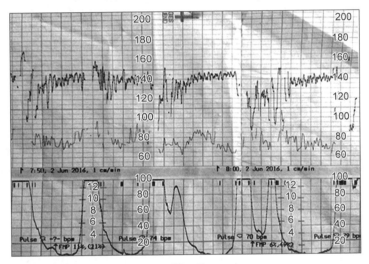

Fig. 6

Questions

1. What is the interpretation of this CTG?
2. What could be the cause?
3. What should be done?

Answers

1. The interpretation of this CTG is:
   - Heart rate is 140 bpm
   - Beat to beat variability is 5–15
   - Recurrent variable decelerations (peak of the deceleration is variable in relation to the peak of uterine contraction)
2. Cord compression, meconium-stained liqor (MSL), and fetal hypoxia
3. If early in labor—plan for emergency cesarean, if during second stage—hasten the process of delivery (instrumental delivery).

Case 4

A 28-year-old primigravida mother diagnosed with gestational diabetes in this pregnancy. She is managed with high doses of insulin at 36 weeks for control of blood sugars. She presented with complaints of pain abdomen for 4 hours. Her admission CTG showed the following pattern (Fig. 7)

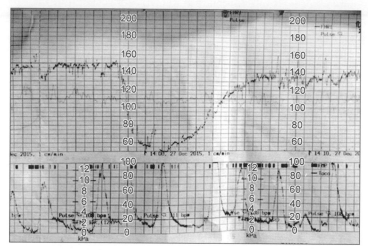

Fig. 7

Questions

1. What is the baseline fetal heart rate?
2. Name the abnormality in the CTG.
3. What is the expected outcome of the baby at birth?
4. What is the expected cord pH?
5. What are the other complications expected in this fetus?

Answers

1. Baseline heart rate is 150 bpm
2. Prolonged deceleration (the fetal rate is at 60 bpm and bradycardia is persisting way beyond the peak of the uterine contraction) and fetal heart rate is falling to 60 bpm for than 2 minutes
3. Perinatal asphyxia
4. pH less than 7.2
5. Subgaleal hemorrhage, intracranial hemorrhage (ICH), caput, and cephalhematoma.

DENVER DEVELOPENTAL SCREENING TEST-II
INTERPRETATION OF REPORTS

Case 1

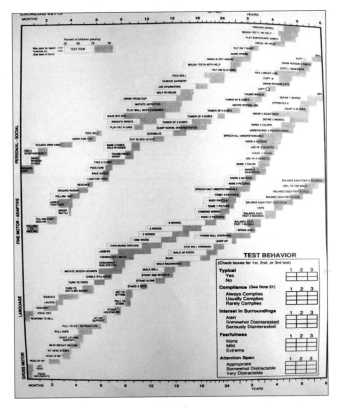

Fig. 8

Questions

1. Identify the above chart (Fig. 8).
2. Till what age can it be used?
3. Till what age do you use corrected age?
4. When to administer to the high-risk newborn (at what all ages)?

Answers

1. Denver development screening test-II (DDST-II)
2. 0–6 years
3. 2 years
4. Corrected 4 months, 6 months, 8 months, 1 year, yearly till 6 years.

Case 2

This chart is used in the assessment of development of a high-risk newborn in the follow up clinic (Fig. 9).

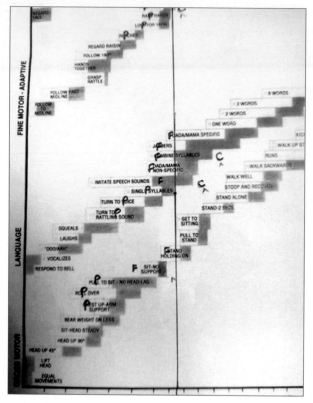

Fig. 9

Questions
1. What do P, F, C, NO, and R stand for?
2. What does the red-colored area represent?
3. What does the vertical line represent?

Answers
1. P—pass, F—fail, C—Caution, NO—no opportunity, R—refusal
2. A delay item
3. Corrected age line.

Case 3

This development assessment on a 8-month-old (corrected age) infant born at 28-week with a birth weight of 1.1 kg.

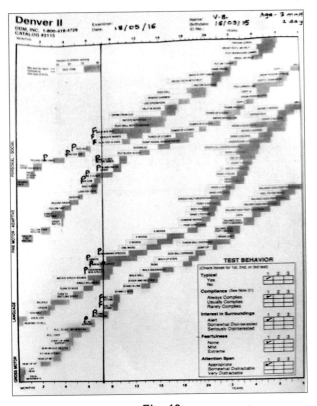

Fig. 10

Questions

1. Interpret the above DDST-II (Fig. 10).
2. What action will you take?

Answers

1. Normal development for age on all four sectors
2. Routine follow up advised.

Case 4

This developmental assessment was done on a high-risk infant at a corrected age of 7 months and 16 days.

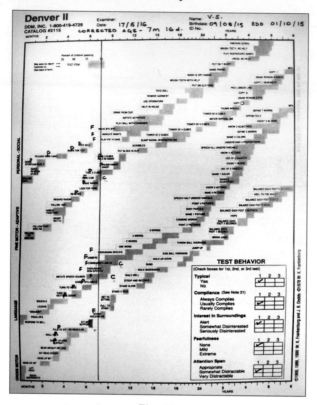

Fig. 11

Questions

1. Interpret the above DDST- II (Fig. 11).
2. What action will you take?

Answers

1. Three cautions and 1 delay: Development is reported as suspect
2. The action points are:
   – Retest in 1–2 weeks if suspect or untestable
   – Refer for developmental assessment scales for Indian infants (DASII) and Neuromotor evaluation
   – Commence early intervention.

NEONATAL ELECTROENCEPHALOGRAM

Introduction

Electroencephalography (EEG) is used as an important tool for assessing neonatal cerebral function, despite the evolution of newer technologies. Though, it is one of the oldest tests, never the less, it is a very valuable tool used for establishing diagnosis and prognosis in some of the neurological conditions, especially in critically ill babies. It is considered more efficient as a predictive test than a neurological examination. However it should always be interpreted in the clinical context and with awareness of the corrected gestational age of the baby.

Describing Neonatal EEG

Before we go on to look at some EEG patterns, it is important to remember certain points:

- EEGs should be interpreted in the clinical context. Always enquire corrected gestational age and the state of the child at the time of the record (awake, active sleep, or quiet sleep)
- Please be familiar with the terms used to describe neonatal EEGs. Assess the EEG in a systematic manner
- First of all start assessing the background activity in all three states wake and sleep (active and quiet sleep)
  - Continuous vs discontinuous
    If discontinuous, calculate the duration of bursts and inter burst interval
  - Inter-hemispheric synchrony vs asynchrony
  - Symmetry
  - Assess the approximate amplitudes in micro-volts
  - Sharp waves are seen in every EEG. Normal or abnormal depends on their abundance and distribution.

It is always important to be familiar with normal EEG for a term infant before going on to identify abnormal patterns

Case 1

A term newborn (3 kg at birth) with birth asphyxia requiring extensive resuscitation is admitted to the neonatal intensive care unit (NICU). He is noted to have clinical seizures at 3 hours and an EEG done at 8 hours of life is shown below (Fig. 12).

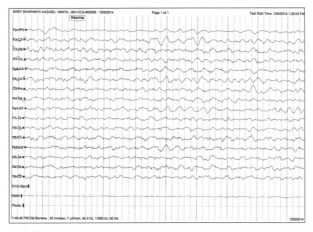

Fig. 12

Questions

1. Describe the findings on the EEG in terms of:
   - Continuous/discontinuous
   - Synchronous/asynchronous
   - Symmetry
   - Sharp waves
   - Amplitudes
2. What is the impression of the background activity?
3. Does the EEG show any seizure activity?

Answers

1. The findings on the EEG are:
   - It is a continuous record
   - It is synchronous
   - There is bilaterally symmetry
   - Occasional sharp waves, predominantly in frontal regions. These are considered sharp transients
   - Borderline amplitudes between 10 and 25 microvolts. In EEGs that are continuous, please look at the amplitudes of the waveforms. The normal amplitudes in awake and active sleep state is between 25 and 50 microvolts. Low voltage: 5–10 microvolts.
2. The background activity is normal and hence the prognosis is going to be favorable
3. There is no obvious seizure activity. This is electroclinical disassociation.

Case 2

EEG of a term newborn presenting with encephalopathy is shown below.

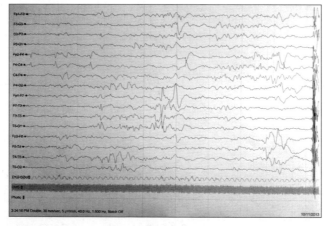

Fig. 13

Questions

1. Comment on the continuity and synchronous status of the above EEG (Fig. 13)?
2. What is the chronology of appearance of synchrony on the EEG in preterm infants?

Answers

1. The EEG of this neonate is discontinuous and is asynchronous (Synchrony: simultaneous appearance of rhythmic pattern over different regions on same side or both sides. Has to be observed in all states (awake, active sleep and quiet sleep)
2. Synchrony starts appearing from 31 to 33 weeks, initially in active sleep. It appears in awake state by about 34 weeks and in quiet sleep by about 36 weeks and beyond.

Case 3

This is the EEG (Fig. 14) of a term newborn (in quite sleep) who had seizures on the first 2 days of life and had required resuscitation with bag and mask for 2 minutes.

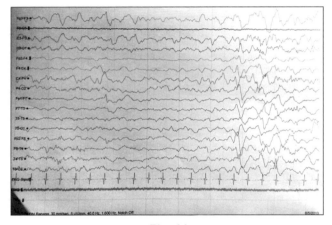

Fig. 14

Questions

1. Comment on the continuity, synchronicity and symmetry of the EEG.
2. What is the diagnosis if this is term baby?
3. What are the possibilities of this pattern if it occurs in preterm infants?

Answers

1. The EEG is discontinuous, synchronous, and there is symmetry
2. Baby is term and in quiet sleep, hence this pattern is called trace alternans
3. Discontinuous EEGs: There are three patterns that one needs to be aware of when faced with discontinuity—trace alternant, trace discontinue and burst suppression. Corrected gestational age and the state of the child are taken into account when interpreting this EEG:
   - Trace alternans–occurs in term babies in quiet sleep. Inter-burst interval has voltages in the range of 10-50 microvolts
   - Trace discontinue: occurs in preterm babies, variable inter-burst interval (depending on the corrected gestational age) and inter-burst voltages ranging from 0 to <25 microvolts
   - Burst suppression pattern: an alternating pattern of high voltage bursts and periods of complete inactivity (voltages of 0 to <5 microvolts) in the inter-burst interval.

Case 4

This is the EEG in a preterm infant who had seizures on day 3 of life (Fig. 15).

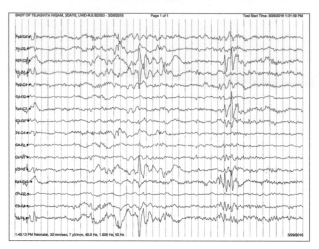

Fig. 15

Questions

1. Comment on the continuity, synchrony, and symmetry of the EEG.
2. What is the diagnosis?

Answers

1. EEG is showing discontinuity. There is synchrony and asymmetry is seen bilateral temporal region (left more than right)
2. Trace discontinue: occurs in preterm babies, variable inter-burst interval (depending on the corrected gestational age) and voltages in the inter-burst interval range from 0 to <25 microvolts.

Case 5

This EEG (Fig. 16) was taken in a term newborn who had refractory seizures.

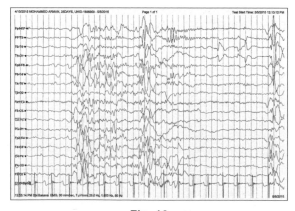

Fig. 16

Questions

1. Comment on the continuity of the EEG.
2. Is there a seizure activity on the EEG?
3. What is the comment on the background activity?

Answers

1. EEG is showing a discontinuous pattern
2. Yes, there is seizure activity on the EEG. There are bursts of high amplitude discharges
3. The background is suggestive of burst supression pattern (generalized bursts of high amplitude discharges with periods of inactivity (<5 microvolts) in the inter-burst intervals).

Case 6

A newborn is admitted to the NICU with encephalopathy and seizures on day 19 of life. A EEG done is shown here (Fig. 17).

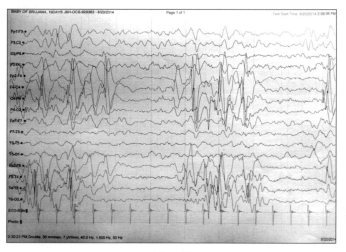

Fig. 17

Questions

1. Comment on the symmetry and continuity.
2. What is the abnormality?
3. Where can you see the abnormality?

Answers

1. This is a discontinuous EEG and with asymmetry
2. High amplitude bursts in the right-sided leads followed by periods of suppression in the inter-burst interval (amplitudes <5 microvolts)
3. The abnormality is seen in all the right-sided leads.

Case 7

Baby A is late preterm infant delivered at 36 weeks by emergency section for decreased fetal movements. The baby did not cry at birth and required extensive resuscitation. The newborn is noted to have early onset seizures, is comatose, hypotonic and on minimal ventilatory support for poor respiratory efforts. Temperature is 36.4°C and blood sugars are repeatedly normal. An EEG of this newborn is shown here (Fig. 18). The newborn is not on any sedatives.

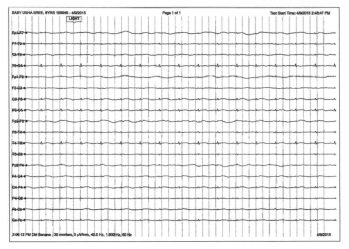

Fig. 18

Questions

1. Comment on the EEG activity?
2. What else need to done to declare the newborn is brain dead?
3. What is the activity that is seen on the EEG due to?

Answers

1. The EEG is showing electro-cerebral inactivity. Voltages <2 microvolts, not reactive to stimuli
2. Brain dead is declared by doing the following:
   - Ruling out hypothermia, hypotension, medications, and other reversible metabolic causes
   - No purposeful response to external stimuli (coma)
   - Absent brainstem reflexes (pupillary, corneal, vestibulo-occular) and gag
   - Apnea test: $PaCO_2$ should increase >20 mm of Hg above baseline and reach at least 60 mm of Hg with no respiratory effort seen
   - Two examinations performed 24 hours apart by two different physicians. Each time an apnea test should be performed
   - EEG done at 48 hours intervals for term and for 72 hours intervals for preterm is just an ancillary test and a definite requirement
3. The activity on the EEG is due to ECG artifacts

Case 8

A term infant with a birth weight of 3.2 kg is discharged on day 3 of life on exclusive breastfeeds. Got readmitted on day 10 of life with poor feeding, lethargy and decreased activity. He is noted to seizures. Admission blood sugar was 20 mg/dL. The seizures continued on day 1 and day 2 of admission. The infant was managed with glucose insulin rate (GIR) of 12 mg/kg/min and multiple anticonvulsants. EEG is shown below (Fig. 19).

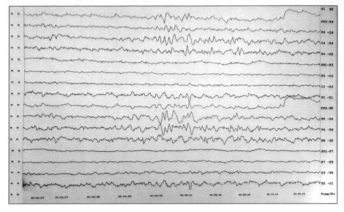

Fig. 19

Questions

1. What is the finding on the EEG?
2. What is the expected long-term outcome in this newborn?
3. What is expected finding on the magnetic resonance imaging (MRI) in this newborn?

Answers

1. Focality is noted in the temporoparietal and occipital regions bilaterally. This insult is most likely due to hypoglycemic brain injury
2. The newborn is likely to have abnormal neurodevelopment and spastic cerebral palsy (CP)
3. MRI in this newborn would show hyperintense signals in the parieto-occipital regions on diffusion weighted imaging (DWI), fluid attenuated inversion recovery (FLAIR) and T2 sequences.

Case 9

Below is the EEG recording of a term newborn who presented with refractory focal seizures (Fig. 20).

Questions

1. What is the abnormality noted on the EEG?
2. What is the most likely reason for this finding?
3. What is an electrographic seizure in a newborn?
4. Should we treat an electrophic seizure in a newborn?

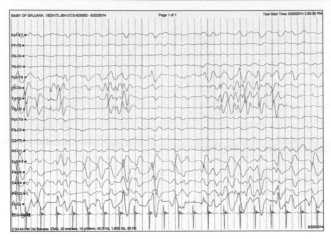

Fig. 20

Answers

1. Continuous spike and slow wave discharges in the right-sided leads. Duration >10 seconds
2. This could be seen with cortical malformation or with an infarct
3. Electrographic seizures: An epileptic phenomenon in the EEG without clear clinical manifestation. Epileptic activity lasting >10 seconds
4. All electrographic seizures in neonates need to be treated.

Case 10

A preterm infant born at 33 weeks of gestation and birth weight of 2.2 kg is admitted to the NICU on day 25 of life with history of lethargy, decreased activity and recurrent apneas. There is a history that many in the family are affected with symptoms of flu. Baby on examination had HR of 152/min, RR of 55/min, CFT normal, mild hepatomegaly, sensorium is depressed, tone is markedly reduced and reflexes are diminished. Baby is on supportive ventilation. Venous blood gas (VBG), ammonia and lactate are normal. Evaluation for sepsis is normal. An EEG done in the newborn is shown here (Fig. 21).

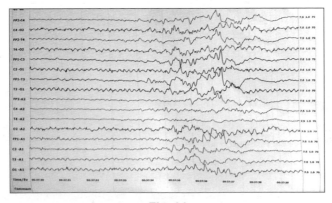

Fig. 21

Questions

1. Comment on the continuity and synchrony of the EEG?
2. What and where are the abnormal discharges?
3. What is the most likely diagnosis?
4. What is the ideal therapy?

Answers

1. The EEG is discontinuous, but has synchronous background in awake state and active sleep
2. Continuous unifocal discharges in the occipital regions bilaterally, lasting > 10 seconds, constitutes electrographic seizures. The 30-minute record had these discharges throughout and was diagnosed as electrographic status. Unifocal discharges of >/= 10 seconds and of any waveform (alpha/beta/ delta) are also categorized as electrographic seizures
3. The most probable diagnosis is herpes simplex virus (HSV) encephalitis
4. The ideal therapy is supportive care and acyclovir for 14 to 21 days.

Case 11

This is the EEG of a 25 day-old baby presenting with refractory seizures (Fig. 22).

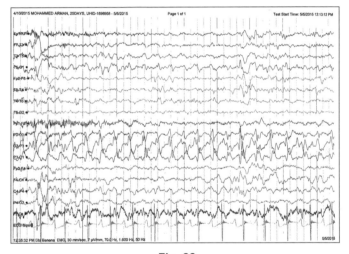

Fig. 22

Questions

1. What is the abnormality seen on the EEG?
2. What are the epileptic patterns on EEG?

Answers

1. Electrographic seizures lasting more than 10 seconds in the left centro-parietal and occipital leads
2. The epileptic patterns (with normal background)
   - Unifocal trains >/= 5 seconds of sharp waves
   - Unifocal periodic lateralized epileptiform discharges (PLEDS)
   - Unifocal discharges of >/= 10 seconds can be of any wave form, alpha/beta/delta.

GENETICS

Accurate documentation of the family history is an essential part of genetic assessment. Family pedigrees are drawn up and relevant medical information on relatives sought. There is some variation in the symbols used for drawing pedigrees. Some suggested symbols are shown in the Figure.

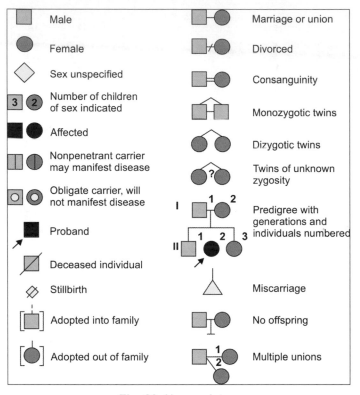

Fig. 23: Nomenclature

Case 1

Newborn baby has flat facial profile, up slanting palpebral fissures, excess skin on back of neck, low set ears. Baby investigated with the following (Fig. 24).

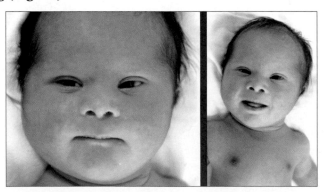

Fig. 24

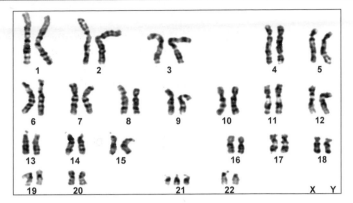

Fig. 25

Questions

1. Is there any abnormality (Fig. 25)? If so what is it?
2. What is the reason behind this abnormality?
3. What are the types of this condition?
4. Is parental karyotype indicated?
5. Is there any recurrence in siblings?

Answers

1. Karyotype, yes; Trisomy 21
2. Down syndrome; Meiotic nondisjunction
3. Three types—Nondisjunction, Robertsonian translocation, and mosaicism
4. Not indicated for pure trisomy (nondisjunction) and mosaic Down syndrome. Essential if translocation or other rearrangement is identified
5. Recurrence risk is affected by maternal age and parental germline mosaicism and type of Down syndrome.

Case 2

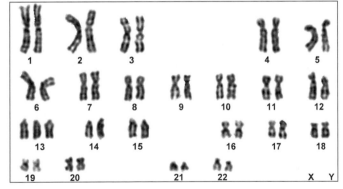

Fig. 26

Questions

1. What is this condition (Fig. 26)?
2. What is the cause?
3. What are the clinical features?

Answers

1. Trisomy 13 or Patau syndrome
2. Approximately 90% are due to non-disjunction in maternal meiosis 1
3. Growth retardation, holoprosencephaly, microphthalmia/anophthalmia, cleft lip and palate, cardiac malformations, postaxial polydactyly, omphalocele, severe mental retardation.

Case 3

Family history of Marfan syndrome (Fig. 27).

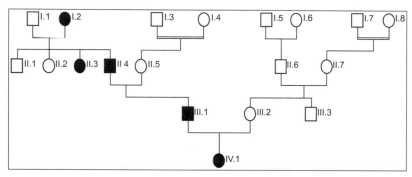

Fig. 27

Question

What is the mode of inheritance? And what are the rules of this inheritance?

Answer

It is autosomal mode of inheritance: Rules of AD inheritance:

• Appears in both sexes with equal frequency
• Both sexes transmit the trait to their offspring
• Does not skip generations
• Affected offspring must have an affected parent unless they possess a new mutation.

Case 4

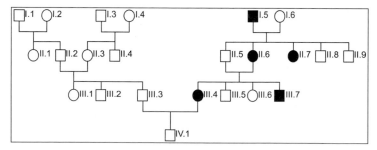

Fig. 28

Question

What is the mode of inheritance in the following pedigree and its rules (Fig. 28)?

Answer

- X-linked dominant pedigree
- **Rules of X-linked dominant**
  - Both males and females are affected; often more females than males are affected
  - Females are less severely affected than males
  - Does not skip generations
  - Affected sons must have an affected mother
  - Affected daughters must have either an affected mother or an affected father.

Case 5

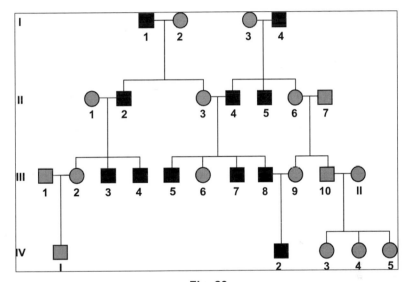

Fig. 29

Question

What is the mode of inheritance and its rules (Fig. 29)?

Answer

Y-linked dominant disorder

Rules for Y-linked dominant

- Only males are affected **NEVER** in females
- It is passed from father to all sons
- It does not skip generations.

Case 6

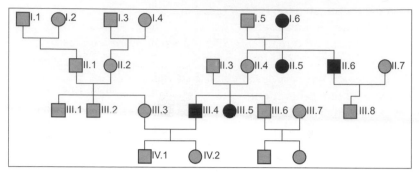

Fig. 30

Question

What is the mode of inheritance (Fig 30)? What the characteristic features of this inheritance pattern?

Answer

Mitochondrial mode of inheritance. The features of mitochondrial inheritance are:

- Trait is inherited from mother only (Matrilineal inheritance)
- Males do not transmit mitochondrial inherited disorders
- Mitochondrial inherited condition can affect both sexes
- Homoplasmy: All copies of mitochondrial DNA have the same sequence (normal individuals)
- Heteroplasmy: Mixture of normal and mutant sequence within same cell (Mitochondrial disorders)
- Percentage of mutant DNA may vary between different tissues and also change with time
- Preferential accumulation of mutant mitochondrial DNAs in affected tissues appears to explain the progressive nature of mitochondrial disorders
- Varieties of mutations occur in mitochondrial disorders (Deletions, duplications and point mutations)
- Point mutations are commonly maternally inherited while deletions and duplications are most often sporadic
- Examples: MELAS (Mitochondrial encephalomyopathy, lactic acidosis and stroke)
  MERRF (Myoclonic epilepsy with ragged red fibers)
  NARP (Neurogenic, ataxia, and retinitis pigmentosa)

Reference Material

Autosomal Dominant Inheritance (Figs 31 and 32)

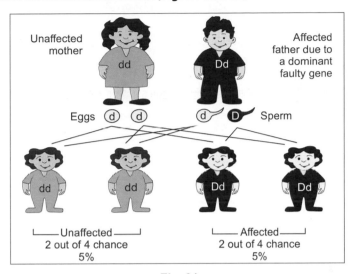

Fig. 31

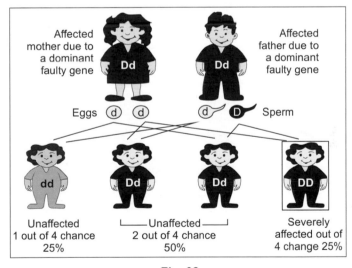

Fig. 32

Autosomal Recessive Inheritance (Figs 33 and 34)

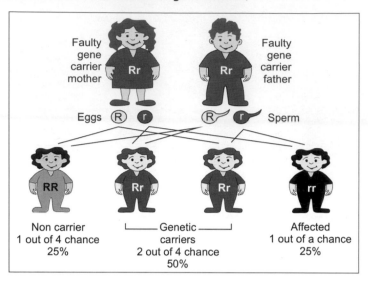

Fig. 33

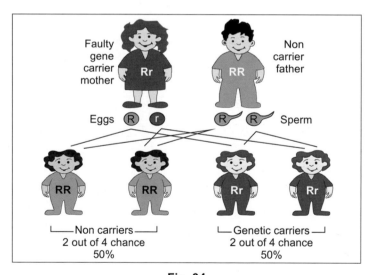

Fig. 34

X-Linked Recessive (Figs 35 and 36)

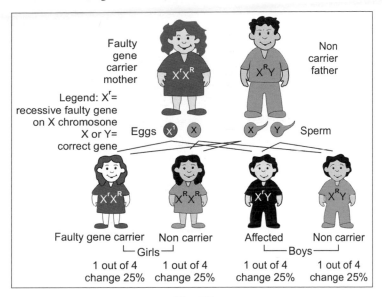

Fig. 35

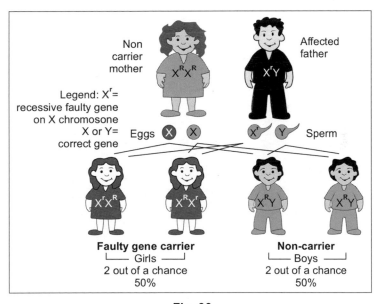

Fig. 36

X-Linked Dominant Inheritance (Figs 37 and 38)

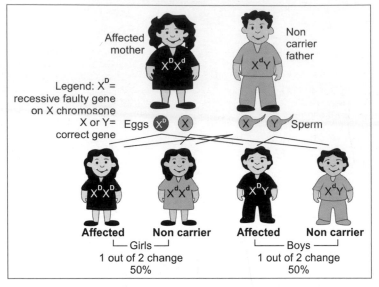

Fig. 37

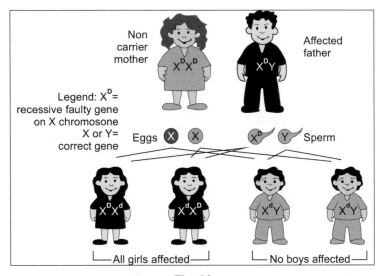

Fig. 38

Mitochondrial Inheritance (Fig 39)

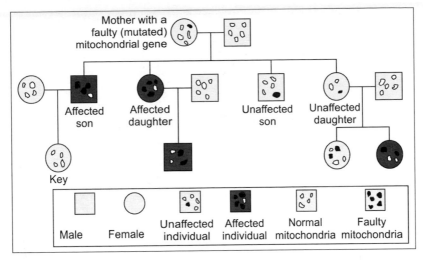

Fig. 39

INTRAUTERINE GROWTH CHART

Case 1

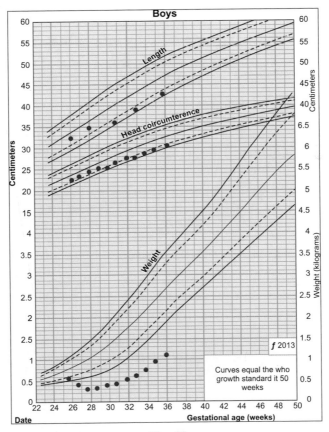

Fig. 40

Questions

1. Interpret the weight for gestational age at birth, and describe in relation to weight at discharge at 36 weeks PMA (Fig. 40)
2. Describe the advantage and disadvantage in using IU growth charts for monitoring postnatal growth of preterm neonates.

Answers

1. The neonate was 26 weeks gestation at birth and weight was on 10th centile. Thus the neonate was appropriate weight for gestational age at birth (AGA). At discharge, weight is far below 3rd centile for 36 weeks PMA. This is interpreted as extrauterine growth restriction (EUGR).
2. Advantage of intrauterine (IU) growth charts: Growth of preterm babies up to term age should ideally follow the trajectory of a normal intrauterine fetus of corresponding gestational age, IU charts provide the best available reference ranges for gestational age. These were obtained from live born neonates delivered at those particular gestational ages (reference charts).

The disadvantages of intrauterine (IU) Charts are:

– The growth ranges are only "reference values" and not ideal standards, as fetuses delivered preterm may not represent a totally normal fetus. Prematurity itself may mean a pathological pregnancy
– The initial days of a preterm neonate is bound to be associated with physiological weight loss that is not corresponding to fetal growth in the same period where there is no "dip" in growth at any point. Trying to emulate this kind of growth invariably results in fluid overload and its possible complications.

HEPATOBILIARY CASE STUDIES

Case 1

Interpretations of investigations in neonatal cholestasis: Differences between cholangiopathy and neonatal hepatitis

	Cholangiopathy	Neonatal hepatitis
Liver function tests	Alkaline phosphatase ↑ GGT ↑ *(Predominant)	SGOT ↑ SGPT ↑ (Predominant)
Ultrasound abdomen	• Triangular cord sign • Gallbladder length <1.9 cm • CBD not seen • Right hepatic artery diameter >1.5 mm • Right portal vein >0.45 • Hepatic subcapsular flow + • Choledochal cyst	- Normal Seen Right hepatic artery <1.5 mm <0.45 - (negative) No
HIDA	No biliary excretion in small intestine	Biliary excretion noted

Contd...

Contd...

Liver biopsy:	• Bile duct proliferation • Bile plugs in ducts • Lymphocytic infiltrates in portal tract	• No bile duct proliferation • Distorted hepatic lobular architecture • Hepatocellular necrosis

* (GGT is normal in PFIC I/II and some IEM of bile acid metabolism)

Abbreviations: GGT, Gamma-glutamyl transpeptidose; SGOT, serum glutamin oxaloacetic transamainase; SGPT, serum glutamiy pyruvic transaminase, CBD, comon bile duct, HIDA, hepatic iminodiacetic acid.

Case 2

Interpret the clinical picture

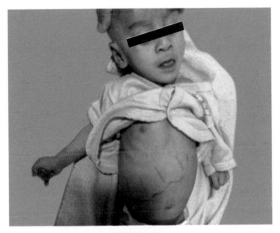

Fig. 41

Questions

1. What is clinical diagnosis (Fig. 41)?
2. What liver pathology is associated with it?
3. What cardiac abnormalities are associated within?
4. What ophthalmic abnormalities are associated with it?
5. Name the vertebral defect associated with this condition.
6. Which gene is implicated?

Answers

1. Alagille's syndrome (broad, prominent forehead, deep-set eyes, and a small, pointed chin)
2. Paucity of bile duct
3. Peripheral pulmonary stenosis, tetralogy of Fallot (TOF), atrial septal defect (ASD), ventricular septal defect (VSD)
4. Posterior embyotoxon, microcornea, optic disk, drusen, shallow anterior chamber
5. Butterfly shape of the bones of the spinal column (vertebrae)
6. Mutation in human Jagged 1 gene (JAGI).

Case 3

Question

What are the recommended doses of the following vitamins for neonatal cholestasis?
1. Vitamin A
2. Vitamin E
3. Vitamin D
4. Vitamin K

Answers

1. 2000-5000 IU/day. Aquasol form
2. 50 – 100 IU/day
3. 3 – 5 mcg/kg/day of 25 hydroxy cholecalciferol
4. 2.5 mg – 5 mg every other day

Case 4

Interpret the findings in this Image.

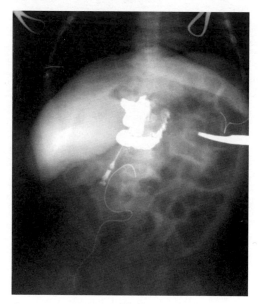

Fig. 42

Questions

1. What is the imaging technique (Fig. 42)?
2. What is its diagnostic significance?

Answers

1. Intraoperative cholangiogram
2. Helps to differentiate neonatal hepatitis from biliary atresia

Case 5

Interpret the image.

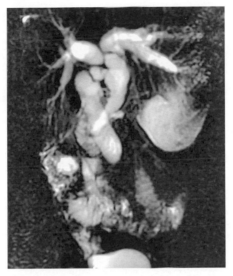

Fig. 43

Questions

1. What is the diagnosis (Fig. 43)?
2. What is the treatment of choice?

Answers

1. Choledochal cyst
2. Hepaticoenterostomy with choledochal cyst excision.

Case 6

Interpret the specimen of ascitic fluid.

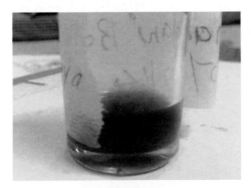

Fig. 44

Questions

1. What is the likely diagnosis (Fig. 44)?
2. What would be serum ascetic albumin gradient (SAAG) in this case?
3. What is the diagnostic test in ascitic fluid to confirm the diagnosis?

Answers

1. Chyloperitoneum
2. SAAG <1.1
3. Ascitic fluid bilirubin >6 mg/dL.

JAUNDICE EVALUATION

Case 1

Using AAP jaundice management chart for phototherapy (Fig. 45)

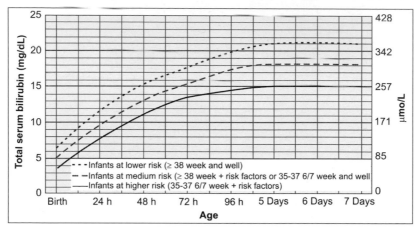

Fig. 45

(*Source:* American Academy of Pediatrics Subcommittee on Hyperbilirubinemia. Management of hyperbilirubinemia in the newborn infant 35 or more weeks of gestation. Pediatrics. 2004;114(1):304).

Questions

1. A cord blood bilirubin of a 8 hours old term infant, 2.5 kg with no risk factors has come as 8 mg/dL. Mother is A Rh –ve and baby is B Rh +ve. How do you use the above chart for management?
2. A day 8 newborn is noticed to be jaundiced on routine evaluation. The baby is well with no systemic signs. The mother is O Rh +ve and baby is A Rh - ve. Total serum bilirubin is 16 mg/dL. How do you plan management using the chart?
3. A day 15 newborn is noticed to be jaundiced on routine evaluation. The baby is well with no systemic signs. The mother is O Rh +ve and baby is O Rh - ve. Total serum bilirubin is 16 mg/dL with direct bilirubin of 5 mg/dL. How do you plan management using the chart?
4. A 36 weeks, well baby, born to primigravida O Rh –ve with baby blood group of A Rh +ve has total serum bilirubin of 15 mg/dL at 36 hours age. What is the best course of action?
5. 38 weeks, 2.4 kg born to primigravida with no risk factors discharged at 25 hours of age is seen with apneic spells at 72 hours. You note jaundice up to thighs. TSB is 14 mg/dL. What is the best course of action: (a) Intensive phototherapy, (b) IVIG, (c) Plan for exchange transfusion, (d) IV Antibiotics with intensive phototherapy, (e) Re-evaluate after 6 hours of intensive phototherapy.

Answers

1. The chart is not applicable in first 24 hours of life
2. The chart is not applicable beyond 7 days of life
3. The chart is not applicable for conjugated hyperbilirubinemia decision making
4. Hospitalize, initiate intensive phototherapy, and re-evaluate TSB after 4–6 hours, assess clinically for signs of encephalopathy
5. (c) Plan for exchange transfusion

Case 2

Using hour specific bilirubin prediction chart

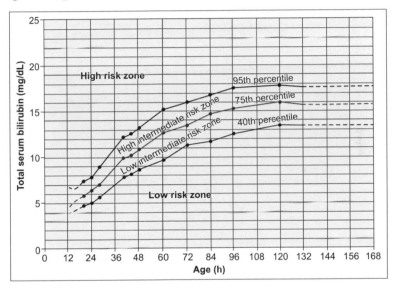

Fig. 46

(*Source:* Bhutani VK, Johnson L, Sivieri EM. Predictive ability of a predischarge hour-specific serum bilirubin for subsequent significant hyperbilirubinemia in healthy term and near-term newborns. Pediatrics 1999;103:9)

Questions

1. You are evaluating a term, 72 hours old, 2.5 kg baby born to mother O Rh +ve and baby blood group A Rh +ve in OPD who appears icteric. The total serum bilirubin has come as 15 mg/dL. What risk zone does this value lie in the above chart?
2. What is the best course of action in the above infant?
3. When do you consider phototherapy in such an infant using the chart?
4. A 72 hours, well baby, born to primigravida, O Rh –ve with baby blood group of A Rh +ve has jaundice up to soles. What it plan of action for this newborn?
5. Baby A has a TSB level of 10 mg/dL at 25 hours of age. Baby B of same age has the same TSB level at 47 hours of age. Which baby is more at risk for severe jaundice?

Answers

1. High intermediate zone
2. Schedule re-evaluation within next 24 hours. If this is not possible keep the baby under observation

3. The chart is not meant for therapeutic decision making. It is meant to identify the potential risk of jaundice and timing of follow up
4. There is severe jaundice. Hospitalize and initiate jaundice management using AAP jaundice charts
5. Baby A

Case 3

Using Tc bilirubinometer chart (Fig. 47)

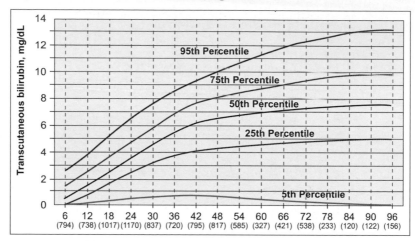

Fig. 47

(*Source:* Maisels MJ, Kring E. Transcutaneous bilirubin levels in the first 96 hours in a normal newborn population of R35 weeks' gestation. Pediatrics. 2006;117: 1170)

1. 34 weeks, 2.1 kg, born to primigravida with no risk factors is found to have Tc Bilirubinometer value of 10 mg/dL at 46 hours of discharge on screening. Mother is O Rh +ve and baby is AB Rh –ve. What it plan of action for this newborn?
2. 36 weeks, 2.4 kg, is found to have Tc Bilirubinometer value of 15 mg/dL at 72 hours of age. What is the next best action you will take?
3. D6 term baby appears icteric up to thighs. Tc bilirubin value is 14 mg/dL. Mother is O –ve and baby is AB Rh +ve. What it plan of action for this newborn?
4. 36 hours, 36 weeks, exclusive breast fed, 2.4 kg has a Tc bilirubin of 10 mg/dL. Mother is AB Rh +ve and baby is O Rh –ve. What is the next best action?
5. A junior resident recommends phototherapy to a 36 weeks, 2.1 kg, with Tc bilirubin of 9 mg/dL at 36 hours of age with Rh incompatibility setting. What is the error in management?

Answers

1. The chart is not applicable for <35 weeks gestation
2. Do a total serum bilirubin
3. The chart is applicable up to 96 hours only
4. Do a total serum bilirubin
5. The chart is not meant for therapeutic decision making. It is a screening tool only

MICRO ERYTHROCYTE SEDIMENTATION RATE

Questions

1. What is the method/procedure of estimation of micro ESR?
2. What micro EST is considered abnormal?
3. What is the sensitivity, negative predictive value of micro ESR?

Answers

1. The procedure of estimation is:
   - Micro ESR is estimated with capillary blood obtained by heel prick, collected in a standard 75 millimeter heparinized microhematocrit tube with internal diameter of 1.1 millimeters
   - Air should not be allowed to interrupt the column of blood to avoid false negative result and one end of the tube should be sealed with 2–3 millimeter of clay
   - The capillary tubes should be anchored firmly with adhesive at the base of the tubes with the names of the patients and time of blood collection stated
   - Alarm clocks to ensure that the one hour sedimentation period is maintained should be used
   - Thereafter, the distance from the highest point of the plasma column to the meniscus of the packed red cell column (height of the plasma column) of each tube was measured with a scale or rule
2. Micro ESR is said to be elevated if the height of plasma column measured is greater than the sum of the age in days and 3 for neonates aged 0–14 days; and greater than 15 mm/hr for neonates aged 15-28 days
3. The sensitivity of micro ESR is around 75% and negative predictive value is 73%. If the micro ESR is combined with band cells will be improved to around 95% and 94% respectively.

NEUROLOGY CASE STUDIES

Case 1

20 days neonate born by normal vaginal birth presented with seizures, frequent tonic spasms with upward gaze and lethargy. There is no history of fever or trauma. On clinical examination the neonate is has depressed sensorium, is hypotonic, Moro reflex is weak. Serum electrolytes, and routine CSF study is normal; metabolic screen is negative. The EEG is shown below (Fig. 48).

Questions

1. Describe the findings on the EEG?
2. What is the diagnosis?
3. What is the investigation required further to confirm the diagnosis?
4. What is the genetic basis for this condition if any?

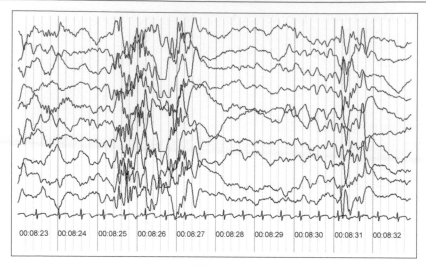

00:08:23 00:08:24 00:08:25 00:08:26 00:08:27 00:08:28 00:08:29 00:08:30 00:08:31 00:08:32

Fig. 48

Answers
1. The findings on the EEG are high voltage bursts (150–300 uV) of spikes or sharp and slow waves, lasting 1-3 seconds with interburst intervals of 3–5 seconds.
2. Ohtahara syndrome (OS)
3. MRI brain to look for structural brain abnormalities
4. The genetic mutations associated with ohtahara syndrome include ARX, STXBP1, SCN2A, KCNQ2, CASK

Case 2

A full term newborn weighing 3 kg at birth and born by assisted vaginal delivery, presented with irritability on day 4 of life. There is no history of fever or seizures or feeding difficulties. On examination the infant had pallor, icterus till abdomen, and no organomegaly. There is a soft fluctuant, nontender large swelling over occipital area extending to temporal and parietal area on both the sides over scalp.

Questions
1. What is the most probable diagnosis.
2. How to differentiate this condition from the other common scalp blood collection?
3. What are the expected complications in this newborn?
4. What is the management in this newborn?

Answers
1. Subgaleal hemorrhage.
2. Subgaleal hemorrhage crosses the suture line while cephalhematoma is restricted to the suture lines
3. The expected complications of subgaleal hemorrhage are:
    - Severe anemia needing blood transfusion
    - Severe jaundice

- Consumptive coagulopathy due ot massive blood loss
- Shock with massive hemorrhage

4. The management is conservative and involves
    - Supportive care
    - Monitoring and management of expected complications

Case 3

Identify the wrong statement regarding therapeutic hypothermia for hypoxic ischemic encephalopathy (HIE).

1. Reduces cerebral energy metabolism
2. Delays apoptosis process
3. Enhances neuronal depolarization
4. Decreases the energy requirement for intrinsic cellular support.

Answer

- Enhances neuronal depolarization

Case 4

Decreased fetal movements are seen in all of the following conditions except:

1. Congenital myopathy
2. Spinal muscular atrophy
3. Duchenne muscular dystrophy
4. Maternal smoking

Answer

1. Duchenne muscular dystrophy

Case 5

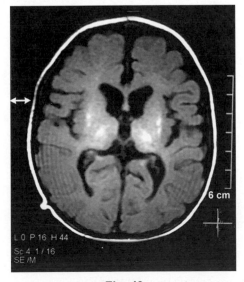

Fig. 49

This is the MRI brain (Fig. 49) of a full-term neonate with an uncomplicated antenatal period. There was history of prolonged labor and meconium stained amniotic fluid.

Questions

1. Describe the findings on the MRI
2. What are the clinical predictors of poor long-term neurodevelopmental impairment in HIE
3. What are the clinical correlates of the findings on the MRI?

Answers

1. Hypoxic ischemic injury to basal ganglia and thalamus
2. The predictors of poor neurodevelopmental outcome are:
   - Initial cord/blood PH <7.0
   - Apgar 0-3 at 5 minutes
   - High base deficits (>-13)
   - Lack of spontaneous activity
   - Decerebrate posturing
   - Refractory seizures, multiorgan dysfunction
   - Absence of spontaneous respiration by 20 minutes
3. The expected neurodeficits are:
   - Dystonic cerebral palsy (CP)
   - Ataxia
   - Bulbar, pseudobulbar palsy
   - Cognitive delay.

Case 6

Antenatal USG at 14 weeks of gestation shows a choroid plexus cyst of 9.5 mm on the right side and there are no other risk factors.

Questions

1. What are the indications for further investigation?
2. What are the associations of these findings?
3. When and What further investigation to be advised?

Answers

1. Isolated cysts are usually benign and most resolve by 24 weeks. However, there is a need to search for other malformations and repeat the scans to assess the size of the cyst
2. The most common associations are trisomy 21 and trisomy 18
3. The furthers investigations in the presence of other major markers or few other markers include:
   - Amniocentesis—karyotype
   - Postnatal neuroimaging

Case 7

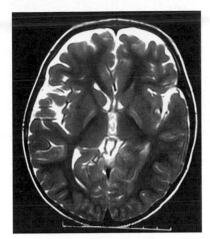

Fig. 50

This is the MRI brain of a full-term, male infant with feeding difficulties and neck retraction (Fig. 50)

Questions

1. What are the findings seen on the MRI?
2. What is the likely etiology
3. What are the expected long-term complications?
4. What is the additional predischarge investigation that helps in identification of etiology?

Answers

1. Hyperintense signals seen in bilateral globus pallidus
2. Kernicterus or bilirubin encephalopathy, mitochondrial disease, or leighs disease
3. Choreoathetoid cerebral palsy, dystonic/dyskinetic cerebral palsy
4. Brainstem evoked response audiometry

Case 8

A day 13 full-term neonate which reported abnormal movements by the parents. There is no history of antenatal or perinatal complications. The infant is feeding well and there is no irritability or lethargy. A small café au lait is noted on the back. Other examination is normal

1. What additional history is required to arrive at the diagnosis?
2. What is the possible diagnosis?
3. What is the expected natural course of this problem?
4. What is the long-term implication?

Answers

1. Movements occurring only in sleep. Mainly in NREM sleep
2. Benign neonatal sleep myoclonus
3. Spontaneous resolution in 2–3 months
4. Normal neurological outcome

232

PARTOGRAPH

Case 1

25 year primigravida at 40 weeks of gestation came with complaints of pain abdomen and is admitted in the labor room, her partograph is as follows (Fig. 51):

Questions

1. Interpret the partograph?
2. What is the duration of active labor? And what happened in this mother?
3. What problems are anticipated in the newborn?

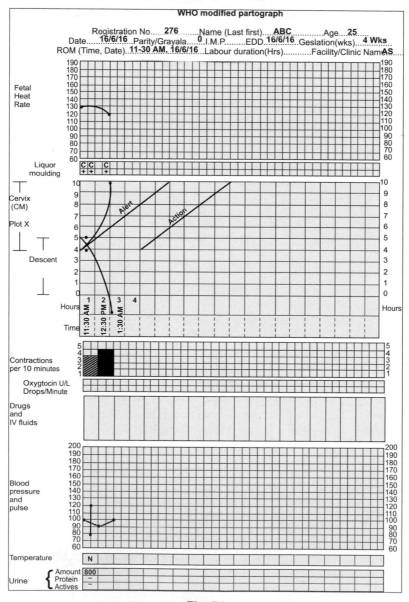

Fig. 51

Answers

1. Full dilatation in 2 hours (expected 1cm per hour), descent of head from 5 to 0 in 2 hours, moderate uterine contractions (lasting for >40 seconds), fetal heart normal and maternal vitals normal
2. 2 hours and precipitate labor
3. Asphyxia, birth injuries such as cephalhematoma and subgaleal bleeds (lack of moulding)

Case 2

25 years gravida 2 para 1 at 39 weeks and 2 days period of gestation presented with history of gestational diabetes. She is admitted in the labor room and her partograph is as follows (Fig. 52).

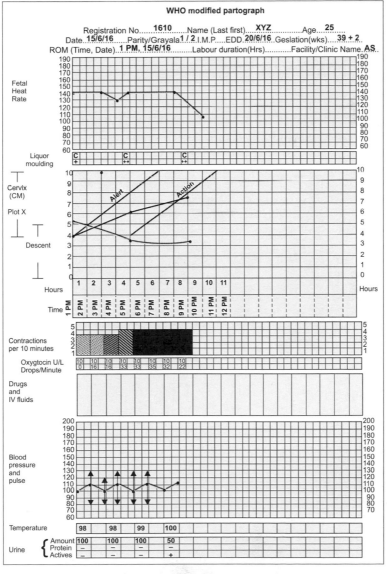

Fig. 52

Questions

1. Interpret the partograph?
2. What are the expected effects on the fetus now?
3. What is the expected course of labor now?
4. What are the complications anticipated in the newborn ?

Answers

1. Change in cervical dilatation of 3 cm in 8 hours, fetal head descent from 5 to 2 in 8 hours inspite of good uterine contractions, fetal heart falling, meconium stained liquor and features of maternal exhaustion (maternal temperature with acetone in urine)
2. Prolonged labor may to fetal hypoxia and fetal acidosis
3. Delivery should be done by cesarean section in view of tardy progress of labor, maternal exhaustion and meconium-stained liquor (MSL)
4. Perinatal asphyxia, persistent pulmonary hypertension (PPHN) and meconium aspiration syndrome (MAS).

PERIPHERAL SMEAR

Case 1

This is peripheral smear of a newborn baby with jaundice on day 1 of life. On examination baby is pale, has icterus, and a palpable spleen.

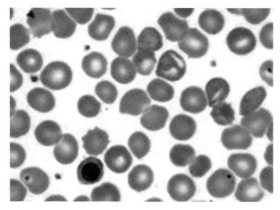

Fig. 53

Questions

1. What are the findings?
2. What are the differentials for these findings?
3. How to differentiate one from the other?

Answers

1. The peripheral smear shows anisopoikilocytosis, polychromasia, burr cells and microspherocytes
2. ABO isoimmunization and hereditary spherocytosis
3. Glucose does not correct the autohemolysis in ABO incompatibility unlike hereditary spherocytosis.

Case 2

This is the peripheral smear of the newborn admitted on day 18 of life with poor feeding, diarrhea, fever, and decreased activity (Fig 54).

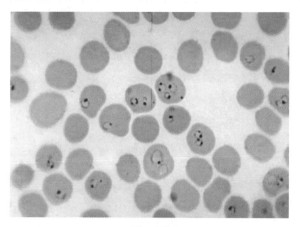

Fig. 54

Questions

1. Identify the smear (Fig. 54).
2. What are the usual manifestations of this problem in the newborn?
3. What is the treatment plan?

Answers

1. Ring stage of *Plasmodium falciparum*
2. Around 80% of the newborn manifest with fever, anemia, and splenomegaly. They can also have jaundice, hepatomegaly, loose stools, and poor feeding
3. Artemisinin-based combination therapy (ACT) is the recommended treatment for uncomplicated malaria in infants.

Case 3

This is the peripheral smear of a newborn presenting on day 9 with off color, decreased activity, periumbilical erythema, and cold peripheries.

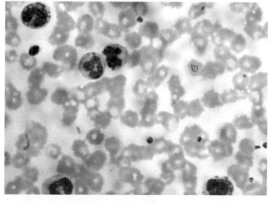

Fig. 55

Questions

1. Identify the smear (Fig. 55).
2. Define the most prominent WBC seen on this smear.
3. What are the parameters taken as significant when a neonate has these findings?

Answers

1. The smear shows presence of band cell, toxic granules, and immature neutrophils
2. Band cell is defined as an immature white blood cell (WBC) with central width atleast 1/3rd of the maximum width of the nucleus of the WBC
3. This indicates a smear of sepsis, the immature to mature ratio of >0.20, toxic granules, shift to left of the leukocytes, more than 20% of band cells are significant.

Case 4

This is peripheral smear of a newborn baby with jaundice on day 2 of life. On examination he was pale, had icterus, palpable spleen. Mother is B-ve and Baby is O - ve.

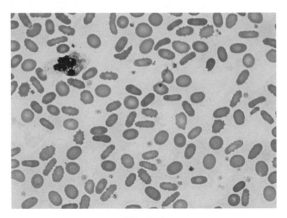

Fig. 56

Questions

1. Identify the smear (Fig. 56).
2. What is the reason for this finding? What are clinical markers for this finding?
3. Can this still be Rh-isoimmunization? Explain.

Answers

1. The smear shows anisopiokilocytosis, polychromasia, pencil cells, and burr cells
2. This finding occurs in hemolysis. The clinical markers are pallor, early and severe jaundice, and splenomegaly
3. Yes, this can still be Rh-isoimmunization. Baby blood group could be pseudo-negative for:
   - After an in utero transfusion with Rh negative blood
   - Prozone phenomenon where all the Rh antigen on the RBC is coated with maternal antibodies and hence a negative blood group

Pulmonary Graphics

Case 1

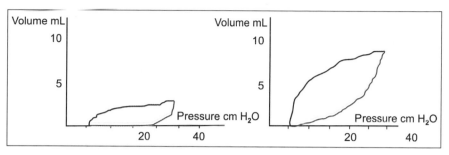

Fig. 57

Questions

1. Describe the change from picture A to picture B.
2. Name 1 intervention that could have resulted in this change (Fig. 57)?

Answers

1. Lower opening pressure, increase in slope and wider hysteresis due to increase in compliance (more volume change for unit pressure change)
2. Surfactant therapy

Case 2

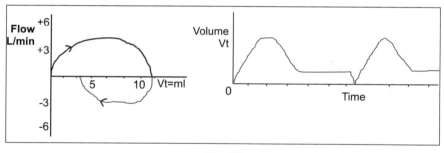

Fig. 58

Questions

1. Describe the graphic represented in the above 2 pictures (Fig. 58).
2. What could be the possible reasons for the above?

Answers

1. (A): Flow volume loop with volume in expiration not returning to zero
   (B): Volume time scalar with volume not returning to baseline
2. Leak due to small ET tube/equipment and circuit leak/high endotracheal tube/faulty calibration of flow sensor.

Case 3

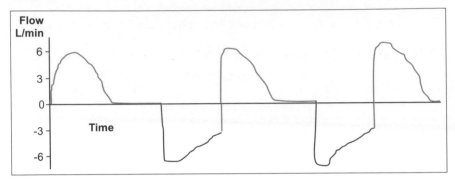

Fig. 59

Questions
1. Enumerate the faulty ventilator settings that could have resulted in this flow time scalar
2. What can be the clinical results of the above?

Answers
1. Unnecessarily long inspiratory time with a period where there is no flow and inappropriately short expiratory time which does not allow expiratory flow to return to baseline, before which inspiration of next cycle commences
2. The clinical effects would include:
   - Exposure to prolonged peak inspiratory pressure (PIP) and
   - Air trapping and hyperinflation—can result in auto positive end-expiratory pressure (PEEP), air leaks, compromised venous return.

Case 4

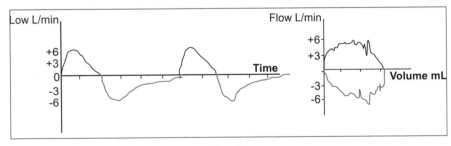

Fig. 60

Questions
1. Describe the above ventilator graphics (Fig. 60)
2. What could be the reasons and what actions are required?

Answers
1. Flow time scalar with drawn-out (prolonged) expiration, Flow volume loop with jagged lines

2. Secretions in endotracheal tube obstructing expiratory flow, and causing irregular flows in both phases of respiration. Suction and clearance of secretions is required. Sometimes even tube change may be warranted

PULSE OXIMETER PREDISCHARGE

Flowchart 6.1

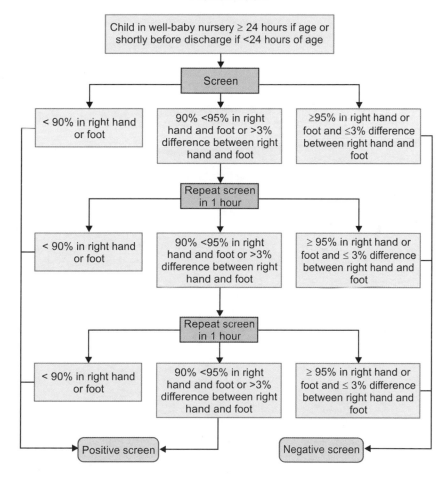

Child in well-baby nursery ≥ 24 hours if age or shortly before discharge if <24 hours of age

Screen

< 90% in right hand or foot

90% <95% in right hand and foot or >3% difference between right hand and foot

≥95% in right hand or foot and ≤3% difference between right hand and foot

Repeat screen in 1 hour

< 90% in right hand or foot

90% <95% in right hand and foot or >3% difference between right hand and foot

≥ 95% in right hand or foot and ≤ 3% difference between right hand and foot

Repeat screen in 1 hour

< 90% in right hand or foot

90% <95% in right hand and foot or >3% difference between right hand and foot

≥ 95% in right hand or foot and ≤ 3% difference between right hand and foot

Positive screen

Negative screen

Questions

1. When pulse oximeter is used as a predischarge screening tool, when is the screening considered positive and what are the interpretations?
2. What are the critical cardiac conditions identified by pulse oximeter?

Answers

1. The screening criteria and the interpretations of a positive screen are:
   - Type 1, universal low saturation: oxygen saturation <90% in either limb on a single reading
   - Type 2, universal borderline saturation: oxygen saturation of 90 to 94% in both limbs on three consecutive readings at hourly intervals
   - Type 3, differential saturation: a difference in the oxygen saturation of 4% or more between the upper and lower limbs on three consecutive readings at hourly intervals

2. Screening by pulse oximeter identifies the following critical congenital heart disease hypoplastic left heart syndrome:
   - Pulmonary atresia
   - Tetralogy of Fallot
   - Transposition of great vessels
   - Truncus arteriosus
   - Tricuspid atresia
   - Total anomalous pulmonary venous return.

SHAKE TEST

Case 1

This test is conducted on a the gastric aspirate of a newborn with birth weight of 1.1kg and gestation of 29 weeks and admitted to NICU with respiratory distress.

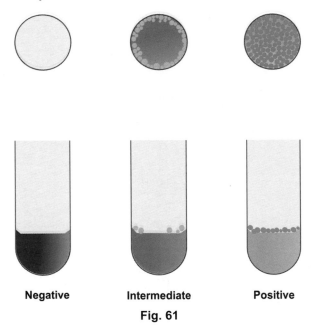

| Negative | Intermediate | Positive |

Fig. 61

Questions
1. What is the test being done and how is it done (Fig. 61)?
2. What is the interpretation of the test?
3. What is the specificity and positive predictive value of this test?
4. What are reasons for a false positive and false negative test?
5. On what principle is the test based?

Answers
1. This is shake test done to assess the lung maturity of the newborn infant. The gastric aspirate taken within 20 to 30 minutes after the delivery (0.5 mL) is mixed with 0.5 mL of absolute alcohol in test tube. This is shaken for 15 seconds and allowed to stand for 15 minutes. The stability of the micro bubbles is observed at the junction of air liquid interface

2. A negative shake test, i.e. no bubbles or bubbles covering less than 1/3rd of the rim indicates a high-risk of developing respiratory distress syndrome (RDS) and the presence of bubbles at more than 2/3 of the rim indicates lung maturity and decreased risk of developing RDS
3. The specificity is 92% and positive predictive value (PPV) is 92–100%.
4. Blood and meconium in the gastric aspirate are the reasons for false positive and false negative shake test
5. Ethanol generates foam in gastric aspirate. All the bubbles will remain intact after 15 minutes if there is surfactant in gastric aspirates.

NEONATAL SURGERY

Case 1

This right cervicoaxillary lesion was diagnosed on the antenatal ultrasound.

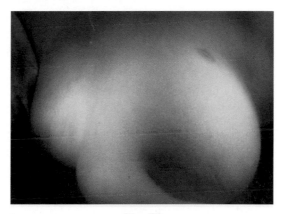

Fig. 62

Questions

1. What is the probable diagnosis (Fig. 62)?
2. What is the natural history of this lesion?
3. State two antenatal/perinatal problem that may arise with large lesions of similar nature.
4. State one neonatal problem that may arise with large lesions of similar nature.
5. Mention two common complications of this lesion causing rapid increase in size.
6. Why is surgical extirpation difficult in many such instances?
7. State one nonsurgical treatment option in selected cases.

Answers

1. Cystic hygroma/lymphangiohemangioma/lymphatic vascular malformation
2. Progressive growth/no spontaneous resolution
3. Hydrops fetalis, obstructed labor, polyhydramnios
4. Respiratory distress
5. Hemorrhage into lesion, infection/lymphangitis

6. The lesion is not well-circumscribed and insinuates between anatomic planes, nerves and vessels
7. Injection sclerotherapy.

Case 2

A 2.5 kg, term newborn presents with abdominal distension, respiratory distress, and drooling of salvia.

Questions

1. What is the most likely diagnosis?
2. What confirmatory test would you do on the bedside?
3. Name 2 other anomalies you would clinically evaluate in suspect esophageal atresia.
4. State any 2 immediate management measures you would adopt.
5. State 2 imaging studies to complete your evaluation.
6. State two factors influencing outcome in EA.
7. Name any two postoperative problem after repair of tracheoesophageal fistula (TEF).
8. Which type of TEF may escape detection in newborn period.

Answers

1. Esophageal atresia or tracheoesophageal fistula
2. Pass a relatively stiff catheter (e.g., rubber) per oral gently to see if it negotiates into the stomach
3. Vertebral, anorectal, cardiac, radial ray/limb
4. Oropharyngeal suction, intravenous (IV) fluids, warming, oxygenation
5. X–ray, infantogram, renal USG, and echocardiography (ECHO)
6. Gestational age/prematurity, cardiac anomalies, and aspiration pneumonia
7. Gastroesophegal reflux (GER), tracheomalacia, and anastomotic stricture
8. H–type TEF.

Case 3

Study the plain abdominal X-ray in a neonate with intestinal obstruction (Fig. 63)

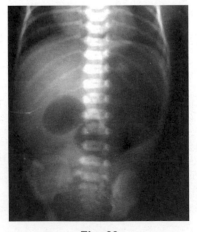

Fig. 63

Questions

1. Describe the classical findings in this X-ray?
2. State one finding on antenatal ultrasonography indicative of upper GI obstruction in the fetus.
3. What pathology is this X-ray diagnostic of?
4. What is the commonest chromosomal anomaly in neonates with these patients?
5. What is the commonest clinical presentation?
6. What type of cardiac defect is associated with cases of this duodenal atresia and Trisomy 21?
7. Which part of duodenum is the usual site of atresia?
8. What is the surgery of choice in duodenal atresia?
9. State two differential diagnosis of duodenal atresia?

Answers

1. Double bubble sign
2. Polyhydramnios, dilated stomach bubble
3. Duodenal atresia
4. Down's syndrome/Trisomy 21
5. Bilious vomiting/bile stained aspirates
6. Endocardial cushion defects
7. Second part
8. Duodeno duodenostomy
9. Annular pancreas, and malrotation of midgut.

Case 4

A male, term neonate did not pass meconium till 52 hours after a normal vaginal delivery. The contrast enema is illustrated in Figure 64.

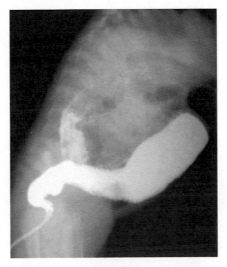

Fig. 64

Sl. No.	Questions	Answers
1	Mention any two notable radiological features in this contrast enema.	• Narrow rectum • Dilated sigmoid colon • Transition zone in rectosigmoid region • Reversal of rectosigmoid ratio
2	What is the probable diagnosis in this case.	Hirschsprung's disease, rectosigmoid type
3	Mention any two common clinical presentation of the disease.	• Neonatal large bowel obstruction • Enterocolitis—sepsis • Chronic constipation, failure to thrive
4	State two differential diagnoses of neonatal Hirschsprung disease.	• Hypoplastic/small left colon syndrome • Meconium plug syndrome • Colonic immaturity in the preterm
5	How is the diagnosis confirmed.	Rectal biopsy, histopathology
6	State two histological features of Hirschsprung's disease on rectal biopsy.	• Absence of ganglion cells in submucous or Myenteric plexus • Hypertrophic nerve bundles in submucosa and lamina propria
7	Name any one definitive surgical procedure in the treatment of Hirschsprung's disease.	• Duhamel's • Swenson's • Soave's

Case 5

This is a male neonate with an imperforate anus (Fig. 65)

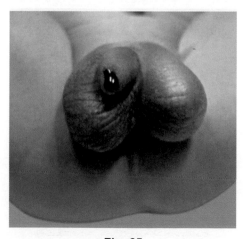

Fig. 65

Sl. No.	Questions	Answers
1	What is demonstrated in this clinical photograph?	Meconuria
2	What is the likely anorectal anomaly in this neonate?	High anorectal malformation, rectourinary fistula
3	What is the currently recommended X-ray to image the level of the malformation? Who has described this radio-graph?	• Cross Table Prone Lateral (Shoot – Through) view • KLN Rao, PGIMER, Chandigarh Invertogram
4	What other gut anomalies would you rule out clinically soon after birth and how?	Esophageal atresia, by inserting a nasogastric tube
5	State two surgical options for high anorectal anomalies.	• Colostomy, then definitive pull – through. • Primary pull through procedure. • Laparoscopic assisted pull through procedure.
6	State two factors that significantly influence the rates of bowel continence after surgery in anorectal anomalies.	• Level of anomaly – high/low • Quality of musculature/sphincters • Number of sacral vertebrae • Technical accuracy of procedure
7	This child has recurrent UTI after all surgical procedures have been completed. Suggest any two possibilities that need investigation.	• Vesicoureteral reflux • Obstructive uropathy • Missed/recurrent rectourinary fistula

Case 6

Study the CXR of this neonate and answer the questions that follow (Fig. 66)

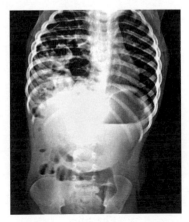

Fig. 66

Sl. No.	Questions	Answers
1	What is the diagnosis?	Right sided congenital diaphragmatic hernia
2	Describe any two diagnostic features on the X-ray.	• Bowel loops in right hemithorax • Paucity of loops in abdomen • Mediastinal shift • Compressed lung
3	Mention any two common clinical presentations.	• Antenatal diagnosis • Neonatal respiratory distress/ cyanosis • Repeated LRTI in infancy
4	What is the commonest associated anomaly?	Congenital heart disease
5	Identify any two abnormalities in the ABG of this newborn? pH – 7.20, $PaCO_2$ – 70 mm of Hg, PaO_2 – 40 mm of Hg, HCO_3 – 16 mEg/l, BE/D –8	• Hypoxia • Hypercarbia • Acidosis, respiratory, partially compensated
6	State two primary steps you would take in the neonatal emergency room as you care for this condition.	• Warming the child • Decompress bowel (nasogastric tube insertion, rectal syringing to evacuate meconium) • Oxygenation
7	On gentle ventilation, there is a sudden desaturation. State any two possibilities.	• Pneumothorax • Ventilator/monitor dysfunction • Endotracheal tube block, dislodgement
8	What are the basic pathophysiological problems in this condition? (Any 2)	• Pulmonary hypoplasia • Pulmonary hypertension • Persistent fetal circulation

Case 7

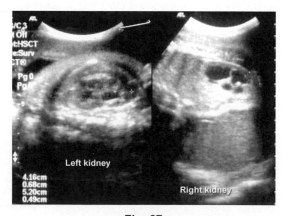

Fig. 67

An antenatal scan in an otherwise uneventful pregnancy at term showed significant bilateral fetal hydronephrosis (Fig. 67)

Sl. No.	Questions	Answers
1	What would you counsel the parents? (Any two)	• Wait and watch • Delivery at tertiary hospital • Reassess at birth • Findings may be normal/pathological
2	You attend this male neonate 24 hours after birth, what would you enquire?	• Voiding pattern • Feeding/general activity
3	What would you look for in a physical examination? (Any two)	• Palpable bladder/kidneys • Spine/anus • Features of sepsis • External genitalia
4	A postnatal USG at 24 hours of birth is reported normal. What is your advice?	• Repeat USG after 72–96 hours of life • Antibiotic prophylaxis till diagnosis is established
5	The repeat USG at 1 week of age is reported as bilateral hydroureteronephrosis. What investigation would you order next?	• Voiding/micturating cystourethrogram (MCUG)
6	State two likely diagnoses in such a scenario.	• Posterior urethral valve • Bilateral vesicoureteric reflux (VUR) • Neurogenic bladder • Ectopic ureter

Case 8

This is a clinical photograph of a female neonate with swelling on the back (Fig. 68)

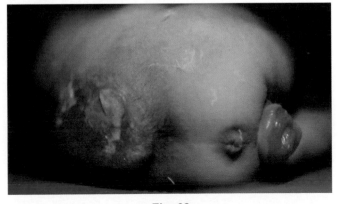

Fig. 68

Sl. No.	Questions	Answers
1	State any two findings on the photograph.	• Spina bifida • Uterine prolapse • Patulous anus
2	State two neurological deficits that are likely in this case.	• Paraplegia • Bowel incontinence • Bladder incontinence
3	An antenatal maternal vitamin supplement is known to decrease the risk of this anomaly. Name the vitamin, its dosage and time of administration.	• Folic acid • 400–500 µg once daily • Preconceptual to 12 weeks gestation
4	Currently, which antenatal imaging can accurately delineate the fetal defect?	Fetal MRI
5	State any two aspects of immediate care you would provide before transferring this to a tertiary care center?	• Occlusive dressing with sterile saline soaked gauze • Systemic antibiotics • Nurse in the lateral/prone position
6	What is the commonest problem associated with or seen after repair of this defect?	Hydrocephalus
7	Name two common causes of congenital hydrocephalus in neonates.	• Aqueductal stenosis • Arnold Chiari malformation
8	State two biochemical estimations which will help in antenatal diagnosis of open spina bifida.	Maternal serum/amniotic fluid Alphafeto protein Amniotic fluid acetylcholinesterase
9	Name any two markers of occult spinal dysraphism.	Lipoma Dermal sinus Hemangioma/vascular mark Tuft of hair/hypertrichosis

9

Observed Station

NEONATAL RESUSCITATION

Demonstrate Routine Care

A term newborn is just born and is crying. There are no risk factors in the mother. How do you assess and manage at birth?

Checklist
• Assess if breathing is well (Yes)
• Postpones cord clamping for atleast 1 minute
• Keeps baby on mothers abdomen. Covers the baby with a dry, clean cloth
• Ensures clear airway, suctions if visible secretions
• Dries the baby, cuts the cord
• Ensures the baby is dry
• Gives to mother for early skin to skin contact
• Asks the mother to initiate breast feeding
• Re-assesses well-being–breathing, activity, feeding.

Demonstrate Positive Pressure Ventilation

A newborn is apneic after initial steps of resuscitation. You may ask relevant details as you proceed to manage this case.

Checklist
• Indicates need for positive pressure ventilation (PPV)
• Calls for help; requests for pulse oximeter
• Positions mask correctly
• Delivers adequate pressure to get chest rise
• Ventilates at appropriate rate (Breathe-two-three to achieve 40–60/min)

Contd...

Contd...

- Requests heart rate (HR) response within 5–10 test breaths

HR....40/min, no breath sounds heard

Takes corrective steps for ventilation
- Reapplies mask
- Repositions baby head
  Assess for chest rise and breath sounds...(No chest rise and breath sounds)
- Suctions mouth
- Ventilates with mouth open
  Assess for chest rise and breath sounds...(No chest rise and breath sounds)
- Increases bag pressure
  (There is chest rise)

Administers effective PPV for 30 seconds

Asks for HR
(HR is 120/min and baby is breathing well)

Gradually discontinues PPV

Demonstrate Management of Meconium Stained Amniotic Fluid Baby

A term, newborn is just born. There is meconium stained amniotic fluid (MSAF). How do you manage in the delivery room.

Checklist
• Asks for respiration, heart rate and tone (baby is not breathing and limp)
• Identifies nonvigorous MSAF
• Cuts the cord immediately and shift the newborn under warmer
• Perform brief and quick oropharyngeal suction (12 G)
• Initiates bag and mask ventilation
• Asks attendant to monitor heart rate
• Looks for chest rise (No chest rise)
• Performs mask readjustment, repositions airway (No chest rise)
• Intubates swiftly for tracheal suction
• Attaches endotracheal (ET) tube to suction machine using meconium adaptor. Applies suction withdrawing ET tube
• Ensures heart rate is rising
• Assess respiration, HR to decide need for further course of action

Note:

a. There is insufficient published human evidence to suggest routine tracheal intubation for suctioning of meconium in nonvigorous infants born through MSAF as opposed to no tracheal intubation for suctioning.

b. The emphasis should be on initiating ventilation within the first minute of life in nonbreathing or ineffectively breathing infants.

c. Appropriate intervention to support ventilation and oxygenation should be initiated as indicated for each individual infant. This may include intubation and suction if the airway is obstructed.

Demonstrate Chest Compression

A newborn has ongoing PPV. There is chest rise but HR after 30 seconds is 50 per minutes? How do you support this newborn.

Checklist
• Indicates need for chest compression
• Asks colleague to electively intubate the newborn
• Ensures 100% oxygen delivery
• Locates the site for chest compression at the lower third of the sternum
• Encircles the chest with hands putting the thumbs adjacent to each other
• Delivers compression with "one and two and three and…" pneumonic followed by a positive breath and ratio of 3:1 with ventilation
• Delivers compression squeezing 1/3 the anteroposterior (AP) diameter of the chest
• Provides uninterrupted coordinated chest compression and ventilation for 45–60 seconds
• Ensures effective ventilation by chest rise
• Asks for HR at the end of 60 seconds

PHENOBARBITAL ADMINISTRATION

You have been instructed to administer injection phenobarbitone to a 3 kg neonate who presented with seizures following hypoxic ischemic encephalopathy. The expected dose is 60 mg. Describe the steps of administration of phenobarbitone to the newborn.

Preparation

- Syringes
- Saline
- Cotton swabs with betadine and spirit
- Needles 24G and 26G
- Infusion pump
- Phenobarbitone injection

Steps of Administration

- Injection comes as a preparation of 200 mg/mL in 1 mL ampoule
- Take 0.1 mL of the solution and dilute it with 0.9 mL of saline
- Calculate the required amount and dissolve in normal saline sufficient to make the total volume 15–20 mL
- Label syringe and attach needle
- Connect syringe to infusion pump
- Set time on infusion pump for 15–30 minutes
- Clean port with spirit betadine spirit
- Start infusion
- Enter in the patient chart dose and time.

UNEXPLAINED BIRTH ASPHYXIA

A 38-week-old male baby is born by normal vaginal delivery. Birth weight—3 kg. The antenatal period and intrapartum period were uneventful. The baby did not cry immediately after birth and required bag and mask ventilation for 2 minutes.

Task: Counseling the parents.

Answers

1. Setting and introduction: Introduces self and greets the informant. Make the family comfortable by offering seats in the counseling room. Informs about what is going to be done
2. Review the history briefly for any missing details of the antenatal and birth and establish rapport (pregnancy details, booking, scan details, occupation and educational status)
3. Inform the current status of the baby
4. Explain to the patient relatives:
    a. Problem of birth asphyxia
        » Birth asphyxia is a common neonatal problem with incidence
        » Immediate risk and the need to monitor—seizures, sensorium, poor feeding, breathing difficulty, urine output, and multiple organ dysfunction syndrome (MODS)
    b. What management is expected?
        » Maintaining temperature
        » Airway and breathing support if any difficulty
        » Intravenous fluids and enteral feeding
        » Blood glucose monitoring
        » Blood tests—calcium level
        » Blood pressure monitoring
        » Monitoring for seizures and seizure control
    c. Possible duration of hospital stay
    d. Estimated cost of treatment
5. Give assurance to the patient's relatives that all possible is being done to improve outcome

6. Inform them few Newborn intensive care unit (NICU) routines such as hand hygiene, visiting policies. Encourage mother to see the baby as soon as possible and talk to the mother directly. Inform about milk expression and colostrum
7. Ask the parents to tell you what they understood
8. Find if they have any more questions. Inform them the time of routine daily counseling and where they can contact you for further clarifications
9. Be polite, compassionate, uses gesture, speaks slowly, clearly, talks less and provokes informant more to speak.

COUNSELING

Admission of a very preterm or VLBW infant into the unit.

Steps

1. Introduce yourself to the parents or guardians
2. Find the details of the mother, father and other relatives and establish rapport (pregnancy details, booking, scan details, occupation and educational status, and contacts with any other doctor or pediatrician)
3. Counsel the parents on the following:
   a. Survival chances (always talk of positive outcomes. It is better to say 70% survival rather than saying 30% mortality). This should be realistic based on the outcomes at your unit
   b. Expected immediate morbidities
      » Respiratory distress syndrome (RDS), need for continuous positive airway pressure (CPAP) and ventilation, need for surfactant
      » Patent ductus arteriosus (PDA) opening on day 2 or day 3
      » Risk of sepsis
      » Nutritional issues (starting feeds, need for colostrum, breastmilk, full feeds and Total parenteral nutrition (TPN)-related issues
      » Intraventricular hemorrhage (IVH) and need to monitor
      » Late onset problems such as retinopathy of prematurity (ROP), necrotizing enterocolitis (NEC), and borderline personality disorder (BPD)
   c. Duration of hospitalization. (clue: Most preterm and VLBW infants are ready for discharge when they reach a gestation of 34 to 35 weeks)
   d. Expected hospital costs
4. Allow the parents or newborn to see their child in the unit with all the support and make them understanding the equipment and their need
5. Encourage mother to see the baby as soon as possible and talk to the mother directly
6. Ask the parents to tell you what they understood
7. Find if they have any more questions.

SUDDEN NEONATAL DEATH IN UNIT

A 2.5 kg girl baby born by normal vaginal delivery (NVD) is found with no respiratory effort and no heart rate in the postnatal ward at 36 hours. The baby was apparently feeding well previously. Despite full resuscitation, the baby could not be revived.

Task: Counseling the family.

Answers

1. Preparation of the setting: Find a quiet room with privacy; encourage spouse/relative to be with father. Greet him and make him comfortable (offer seat) and maintain eye contact throughout the session
2. Introduce clearly with your name and designation
3. Explain why the counseling and ask him what he knew already
4. Use empathetic words/statements, ("I am afraid/unfortunately/I have a bad news") do not falter and after every statement, pause and wait for the father to ask question/express feelings
5. Allow time for the father to respond—express his feelings and ask questions. Listen carefully and this will help in assessment of his reaction to the tragedy
6. Acknowledge and reflect their emotions—observe for any emotion from patient and then respond accordingly. "I understand how this news was a huge shock to you and your family"
7. Reassure the parents that everything possible was done to the baby
8. Be honest and explain that you are not aware of the cause of death. Explain that in sudden cot death, review and certain investigations are required
9. If the family is up to it, review the history (history of maternal and antenatal risk factors and infant risk factors; any symptoms prior to the event). Explain the possible causes for sudden death (infection, sepsis, meningitis, arrhythmias, congenital heart disease (CHD), pulmonary hypertension, aspiration, inborn errors of metabolism (IEM), and arteriovenous (A-V) malformation)
10. Discuss what investigations would be sent (blood for metabolic, septic work-up, postmortem cerebrospinal fluid (CSF) analysis)
11. Assure the family that if they are willing, then autopsy may be done
12. Ask the parents if they want to spend some time with the baby. In case the parents have any special requests like photograph and religious rites, tell them how it can be carried out in NICU
13. Tell them that you would arrange assistance for breast engorgement problem that may ensue
14. Explain in detail the next process involved in taking their young one home and discuss the need for an autopsy if needed
15. Mention the support system available in your institution for bereaved parents. Plan on a future meeting to review the results of the investigations/ autopsy
16. Ask the patient relatives if there is any query. Mention how they can contact you for any further queries in case needed and planning subsequent pregnancies.

SUDDEN DEATH OF A NEWBORN IN THE UNIT

A term 38-week-male baby was born, by emergency low segment cesarean section (LSCS) for placental abruption, with no heart rate and respiratory effort. Despite full resuscitation for 20 minutes, baby could not be revived.

Task: Breaking news to father and helping him handle grief.

Answers

1. Preparation of the setting: Find a quiet room with privacy; encourage spouse/relative to be with father. Greet him and make him comfortable (offer seat) and maintain eye contact throughout the session
2. Introduce clearly with your name and designation
3. Explain why the counseling and ask him what he knew already
4. Allow time for the father to respond—express his feelings and ask questions. Listen carefully and this will help in assessment of his reaction to the tragedy
5. Explain how placental abruption occurs, its nonpredictability and fetal implications in simple language (no medical jargons), build up to the final situation and tell what happened in the end
6. Explain about blood loss due to abruption and ensuing problem to the baby (shock) and how difficult it is to resuscitate in such situations
7. Reassure the parents that everything possible was done to the baby
8. Use empathetic words/statements, ("I am afraid/unfortunately/I have a bad news") do not falter and after every statement, pause and wait for the father to ask question/express feelings
9. Acknowledge and reflect their emotions—observe for any emotion from patient and then respond accordingly. "I understand how this news was a huge shock to you and your family"
10. Do not be judgmental and blame the parents for any of their actions
11. Ask the parents if they want to spend some time with the baby. In case the parents have any special requests like photograph and religious rites, tell them how it can be carried out in NICU
12. Tell them that you would arrange assistance for breast engorgement problem that may ensue
13. Explain in detail the next process involved in taking their young one home and discuss the need for an autopsy if needed.

PREVIOUS SIBLING UNEXPECTED DEATH

Focused History and Examination

History

1. Sequence of events before the death of the newborn
   a. Vomitings, altered sensorium, seizures, fast breathing, rapid deterioration, normal and birth and first 48 hours: Inborn errors a metabolism (IEM)
   b. Decreased activity, dullness, mottled, pallor, fast breathing, cold peripheries, normal at birth and first few days: Duct dependent CHD

c. Well in the first one or two weeks, vomiting, poor feedings, mottled, hyperpigmentation of genitals and axilla, suggestion of electrolyte imbalance: congenital adrenal hyperplasia (CAH)

d. Sudden death: No preceding history or illness: Prolonged QTc

e. Early morning death usually after 4 weeks: Fatty acid oxidation defects or Glycogen storage disorders

2. Examination:
   a. Observation for first few days
   b. Genitals: Hyperpigmentation and ambiguity
   c. Penis size
   d. Soft hepatomegaly and mild tachypnea
   e. Vomiting and not regurgitations
   f. Femoral pulses

3. Baseline tests
   a. Random blood sugar (RBS)
   b. Electrocardiography (ECG)
   c. Newborn screening (acylcarnitine profile)

CONSENT FOR A NEW DRUG OR TRIAL

A 31-week gestational age male baby (B WT 1250 g) born by NVD. Mother was admitted with preterm labor, received one dose of antenatal corticosteroids. At birth, HR < 100/min and he had poor respiratory effort. He was intubated and brought to NICU. He is on 60% FiO_2 and pressure of 20/5. He needs surfactant. Your institute is conducting a randomized controlled blinded trial on two kinds of surfactant.

Task: Consent for a new drug trial

Answers

1. **Setting and introduction:** Seat the parents in a quiet room. Introduce and greet the caregiver

2. **Update on baby:**
   a. Discuss the present condition of the baby
   b. Elaborate on the current standard of care and its limitations

3. **Role of new drug:**
   a. Discuss why a new drug is being considered
   b. The possible adverse effects of the drug

4. **Drug trial: Discuss the following:**
   a. Introduce the drug trial
   b. Chances of either getting the new drug or not (based on the trial design)
   c. The safety system in place for monitoring for adverse effects
   d. Benefits for the family by being involved in the trial (free drug, free treatment, and altruistic for science)
   e. Duration of treatment and the time the baby will be a part of the study
   f. Assure that the study is approved by the Institutional Ethics Committee (IEC) for ensuring that the baby's interests are primary. Discuss rights

to publish. Assure that the privacy and confidentiality of the baby will
always be maintained

   g. Check frequently if the family understands what is being communicated

5. Use simple language without medical jargon. Maintain eye contact
throughout

6. **Patient information sheet (PIS):** Gives time for family to read the PIS in
their language. Encourage queries and clarify

7. **Choice for family:** Ensure the family that they have an option to refuse to
participate in the trial and that they can withdraw from trial at any point.
Assure best possible care at all times irrespective of participation in the
trial

8. **Consent form:** If the parent is willing, get the consent form signed by
investigator and caregiver and witness. Give copy of consent form

9. Ask the parent if there is any query and inform who to contact for any
clarifications regarding the trial

10. Thank and concludes the session.

CONSENT FOR THERAPEUTIC HYPOTHERMIA

**A 38-week-old male baby is born by LSCS. Intrapartum
cardiotocography (CTG) had late decelerations. Birth weight—3
kg. The baby did not cry immediately after birth and required bag
and mask ventilation for 2 minutes. The cord ABG – pH 6.9, PaO_2 – 14,
$PaCO_2$ – 72, HCO_3 – 8, BE – 20. The baby is lethargic, has abnormal
movements suggestive of subtle seizures, dilated reacting pupils,
with reduced spontaneous movements, and poor newborn reflexes.**

**Task: Counsel the parents for therapeutic hypothermia (TH) and
obtain consent**

Answers

1. Setting and introduction: Introduce self and greet the informant. Make the
family comfortable by offering seats in the counseling room

2. Asks the family what they have understood of the situation

3. Listen and ensure that the family is aware of the following:
   a. Present condition of the baby—baby in moderate asphyxia/has seizures
   b. Possible multisystem complications of the problem
   c. Discuss the various modalities of treatment—in vitro fertilization (IVF),
ventilation, drugs for seizures, and various blood tests required
   d. Possibility of long-term neurodevelopmental problems

4. Discuss therapeutic hypothermia (TH)
   a. What is therapeutic hypothermia:
     » Cooling the baby 33°–34°C and maintaining at that temperature
without any fluctuations
     » Core temperature monitoring
     » 72 hours
     » Slow rewarming
   b. Why cooling?
     » Explain about continued reperfusion injury in simple language

   c. How is it done?
- » Ice packs/Miracradle/Tecotherm.

   d. How it helps the baby
- » Reduces adverse neurodevelopmental outcomes by 30%

   e. Side effects (Coagulopathy, bradycardia, subcutaneous fat necrosis)

   f. Monitoring involved:
- » Protocol-based blood investigations/interventions
- » Continuous monitoring of core temperature

   g. Cost

   h. Follow-up schedule and the interventions planned

5. Counseling skills
   a. Check frequently if the family understands what is being communicated
   b. Use simple language without medical jargon
   c. Be polite and compassionate
   d. Appropriate nonverbal communication
   e. Give opportunity for caregiver to raise queries
   f. Answer all the queries clearly and patiently
6. Inform them few NICU routines such as hand hygiene, visiting policies. Encourage mother to see the baby as soon as possible and talk to the mother directly. Inform about milk expression and colostrum
7. Sign consent form by caregiver and treating doctor
8. Thank and inform the caregiver the time of next update/counseling.

DEATH OF ELBW BABY

A 27-week gestational age male baby (B WT 850 g) born by NVD. Mother was admitted with preterm labor and delivered within couple of hours of admission. There was no time to give steroids. At birth, HR <100/min and he had poor respiratory effort. He was intubated and given surfactant, has been ventilated since. He needed high pressures and FiO$_2$ initially but gradually weaned to 40% FiO$_2$ and Pressure of 20/5 on day 3. He was started on TPN via UVC on Day 1 and trophic feeds of 20 mL/kg/day on day 2. On day 3, he suddenly went apneic, bradycardia and looked pale. He was thought to have developed severe IVH (bedside ultrasound showed bilateral large IVH) and full CPR was given including emergency blood transfusion. However, he deteriorated and could not be revived.

Task: Breaking bad news to parents

Answers

1. Preparation of the setting: Give them a quiet space for privacy and encourage family to be present. Greet them, make them sit comfortably and maintain eye contact throughout the session
2. Introduce clearly with your name and designation and explain why you are here. Check their understanding so far
3. Give sufficient time to parents first, let them ask questions and express their concerns. Listen to them carefully without interruption

4. Explain why IVH in preterm babies, how common it is in extreme preterm babies. Also, talk to them about non-availability of any treatment to prevent IVH apart from close monitoring. The language used with the parents should be preferably their own and appropriate to their educational levels. (no medical jargons)

5. Explain about blood loss and ensuing problem to the baby (Shock) and how difficult it is to resuscitate in such situations

6. Reassure the parents that everything possible was done to the baby

7. To facilitate understanding it may help to show concrete evidence such as ultrasound. Please check understanding

8. Show them the baby and the support systems given to the baby

9. Use empathetic words, build trust by clear and consistent information delivered with compassion

10. Summarize and inform the plan of action—explain in detail what happens next/when the baby will be ready for father to take home/what formalities to be completed/discuss the need for postmortem if any

11. Ask the parents if they want to spent some time with the baby

12. Mention that you would see them again for any further queries—later that day/follow-up-OPD appointment for medical and psychosocial follow–up and to plan subsequent pregnancy

13. Inform them that Institutional level and community level support systems are available and you will help them.

DEATH OF A BABY AFTER A PROLONGED HOSPITAL STAY

A 28-week gestational age male baby (body weight 980 g), has been in the unit for 4 weeks. He was born by NVD and needed minimal resuscitation at birth, given INSURE (intubation, surfactant, extubation) and was on NCPAP (nasal continuous positive airway pressure) for 2 weeks. He achieved full enteral feeds by 2 weeks of age and had no sepsis. Until yesterday, he was on no respiratory support, tolerating 180 mL/kg of EBM (expressed breast milk) with full strength fortifier and gaining weight (current weight 1.2 kg). Since yesterday night, he has been unwell with distention of abdomen, bilious aspirates and frequent apneas. He was diagnosed to have NEC, kept nil by mouth, started on antibiotics. However, he deteriorated with discolored abdomen and shock – possible perforation. Despite full resuscitation, he succumbed

Task: Counsel parents

Answers

1. Preparation of the setting: Find a quiet room with privacy, encourage relatives to be with parents. Make them at ease (offer seat) and ensure visual contact

2. Briefly introduce yourself (as they would know you) and break the sad news
3. Allow sufficient time for them to react, grieve, touch the baby and ask questions. Answer questions honestly, give consistent information and face them calmly
4. Tell what happened to their baby the previous night and explain how the baby took a bad turn. Give details about necrotizing enterocolitis how commonly it can occur in extremely premature vulnerable babies in simple language. Explain how devastating it could be
5. Reassure that their baby was given best of care and appreciate them for all the efforts they have put in for their baby
6. Be compassionate and use statements like, "I am sorry/"I wish things would have ended differently/I am sad for you". Assess their response and act accordingly
7. Do not argue with even if emotions ride high with parents and do not say words like "Time will heal"/"It's good your baby died before you got to know him or her well"
8. Pacify and give emotional support if their grief becomes overwhelming and they break. (Quietly you can give a tissue). Tell them how well you understand their profound loss and convey to them that you are ready to extend help of any kind that would alleviate their grief
9. Tell them that you would arrange assistance for breast engorgement problem that may ensue
10. In case the parents have any special requests like photograph and religious rites, tell them how it can be carried out in NICU
11. Explain in detail the next process involved in taking their young one home and discuss the need for an autopsy if needed
12. Mention the support system available in your Institution for bereaved parents and how you would be available for any further queries in case needed and planning subsequent pregnancies

DEATH OF BABY OPERATED FOR DIAPHRAGMATIC HERNIA

Term female baby with antenatal diagnosis of congenital diaphragmatic hernia was born in your unit. She has been in your unit for 6 weeks now. She was born in poor condition with bradycardia and poor respiratory effort. She was resuscitated with intubation and ventilated with high pressures. For first 3 days she was oscillated and needed 100% FiO_2 with NO for PPHN (persistent pulmonary hypertension of the newbirth). She also received maximum inotropic support. On day 4, he responded to the supportive care, hence, she underwent surgical correction for diaphragmatic hernia. Since the surgery, he was weaned from ventilation and extubated on day 10 of life. However, establishing feeds was very difficult as there was feed intolerance. He received TPN via peripherally sited long line. On day 40, he was unwell with frequent apneas and desaturations. He was ventilated, needed high pressures of PIP (peak inspiratory pressure) of 34 cm and FiO_2 100%.

Blood tests showed CRP (C-reactive protein)—248 mg/L, platelets were 80,000. Second line antibiotics were started and long line was removed. However, he deteriorated steadily and died on day 42 because of staphylococcal sepsis and disseminated intravascular coagulation (DIC).

Task: Counsel parents

Answers

1. Preparation of the setting: Find a quiet room with privacy; encourage relatives to be with parents. Make them at ease (offer seat)
2. Briefly introduce yourself (as they would know you) and break the sad news. Anger and hostility may be present in patient reaction and address them calmly
3. Allow sufficient time for their interaction and it should be an open dialogue. Avoid altercations while answering the questions and give factual information
4. Explain in detail about the bad turn of events that led on to the end scenario. Give the details about sepsis, actions taken and how it could be detrimental for life in simple language. The choice of language would be their mother tongue
5. Reassure that their baby was given best of care possible
6. Be compassionate and parents should be approached in a humane way. Judge their response and act accordingly
7. Pacify and give emotional support if they break and start crying. Allow them to express their grief (Quietly you can give a tissue or hold their hands). Tell them how well you understand their profound loss and convey to them that your team is ready to extend help of any kind that would alleviate their sorrow
8. Tell them that you would arrange assistance for breast engorgement problem that may ensue
9. In case the parents have any special requests like carrying out spiritual rites (Photograph, Baptism) tell them how it can be performed in the unit
10. Explain the hospital process involved in taking their young one home and discuss the importance and need for an autopsy in this case as significant new clinical information may emerge
11. Mention the system available in your Institution for early anomaly detection which could be of help in subsequent pregnancies.

10

Miscellaneous

INDIA DEMOGRAPHICS SPOTS

India Newborn Action Plan (INAP) 2014

1. India contributes to 17.5% of world population.
2. India contributes to nearly 1/5 of total live births.
3. India contributes to 16% of global maternal deaths, 21% of under-5 deaths and 27% of neonatal mortality.
4. India accounts for more than 40% of global burden of low birth weight babies.
5. About 30% of annual neonatal births in India are contributed by low birth weight babies. Of these 30%, 60% are born at term after fetal growth restriction and 40% are born preterm.
6. The contribution of neonatal deaths to under-5 mortality is 56% (2012).
7. The estimated stillbirth rate (SBR) is 22 per 1000 live births. (Lancet. 2011).
8. The estimated neonatal mortality rate (NMR) is 29. (SRS Statistical Reports, 2000–12).
9. The estimated extended neonatal mortality rate (ENMR) is 23. (SRS Statistical Reports, 2000–12).
10. The NMR in rural area is twice NMR in urban area (33 vs. 16 per 1000 live births).
11. NMR amongst urban poor (37/1000 live birth) is higher than urban average NMR (29/1000 live births). (NFHS 3).
12. The state with least NMR is Kerala (7/1000 live births).
13. Madhya Pradesh has the highest burden of early newborn deaths (0–7 days) at 32, followed closely by Uttar Pradesh and Odisha (30).
14. Four states, Utter pradesh, Madhya Pradesh, Bihar and Rajasthan, contribute to 56% of total neonatal mortality of India.
15. NMR in India (SRS, 2012).

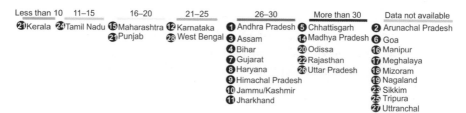

Fig. 1: NMR in India (INAP 2014)

1. Causes of neonatal deaths in India

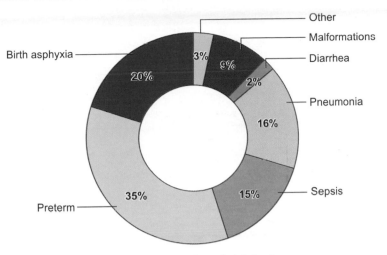

Fig. 2: Causes of neonatal deaths

Source: Liv et al, Lancet, 2012

2. Distribution of neonatal deaths with timing.
   - About 40% of all stillbirth and neonatal deaths take place during labor and within 48 hours of life
   - About ¾th of total neonatal deaths occur within first week of life
   - First 24 hours of life account for 1/3rd (37%) of deaths occurring during the entire neonatal period.
3. The prevalence of birth defects is 6–7%.
4. The common birth defects include congenital heart disease (8–10/1,000 live births), congenital deafness (5.6–10/1,000 live births) and neural tube defects (4–11.4/1,000 live births) (March of Dimes Report, 2006).
5. Interventions Under National Health Mission focusing on newborns:
   a. Janani Suraksha Yojana (JSY), 2005
   b. Integrated Management of Neonatal and Childhood Illness (IMNCI) at community level and F-IMNCI at health facilities, 2007
   c. Navjat Shishu Suraksha Karyakram (NSSK), 2009
   d. Janani Shishu Suraksha Karyakram (JSSK), 2011
   e. Facility-based Newborn Care (FBNC), 2011
   f. Home-based Newborn Care (HBNC), 2011
   g. Rashtriya Bal Swasthya Karyakram (RBSK), 2013
6. The goal of INAP is:
   (a) Ending preventable newborn deaths to achieve single digit NMR by 2030 with all the states to individually achieve the target by 2035.
   (b) Ending preventable stillbirths to achieve single digit SBR by 2030 with all the states to individually achieve the target by 2035.

7. Antenatal care

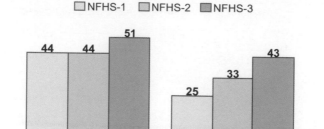

Fig. 3: Antenatal care

Source: NFSH-3, India (2005-06)

8. Delivery care

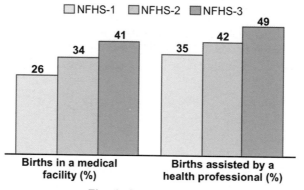

Fig. 4: Care at delivery

Source: NFSH-3, India (2005-06)

9. Mother's age at the time of birth

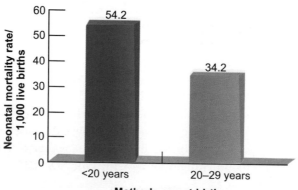

Fig. 5: Mother's age at the time of birth

Source: NFSH-3, India (2005-06)

10. Mortality and birth interval

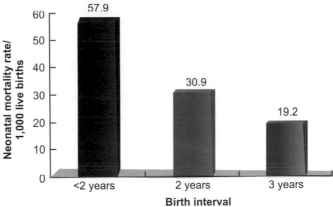

Fig. 6: Birth interval and NMR
Source: NFSH-3, India (2005-06)

11. Mortality and income

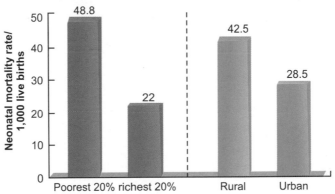

Fig. 7: Income and NMR
Source: NFSH-3, India (2005-06)

12. Mortality with birth size

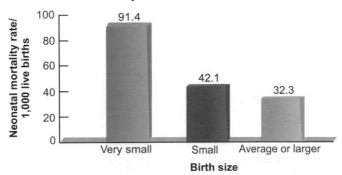

Fig. 8: Size at birth and NMR
Source: NFSH-3, India (2005-06)

13. Institutional deliveries

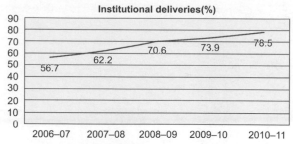

Fig. 9: Institutional deliveries

Source: Family Welfare Statistics, 2010

14. The State of World's Children, WHO, 2012

Countries and territories	Under 5 mortality rank	Under-5 mortality rate		Infant mortality rate (under 1)		Neonatal mortality rate	Total population (thousands)	Annual no. of births (thousands)
		1990	2010	1990	2010	2010	2010	2010
India	46	115	63	81	48	32	1,224,614	27,165

	Annual no of under-5 deaths (thousand)	GNI per capita (US $)	Life expectancy at birth (years)	Total adult literacy rate (%)	Primary school net enrolment ratio (%)	% share of household income 2000–2010*	
	2010	2010	2010	2005–2010*	2007-2009*	lowest 40%	highest 20%
India	1,696	1,340	65	63	97	19	45

Countries and territories	Under-5 mortality rank	Under-5 mortality rate				Average annual rate of reduction (%)				Reduction since
		1970	1990	2000	2010	1970–1990	1990–2000	2000–2010	1990–2010	1990 (%)
India	46	188	115	86	63	2.5	2.9	3.1	3.0	45

	Reduction since	GDP per capita average annual growth rate (%)			Total fertility rate			Average annual rate of reduction (%)	
	2000 (%)	1970–1990	1990–2010	1970	1990	2010		1970–1990	1990–2010
India	27	2.1	4.9	5.5	3.9	2.6		1.7	2.0

15. Evidence-based interventions for mother and child

	Amount of evidence	Reduction (%) in all-cause neonatal mortality or morbidity/ major risk factor if specified (effect range)
Preconception		
Folic acid supplementation	IV	Incidence of neural tube defects: 72% (42–87%)
Antenatal		
Tetanus toxoid immunization	V	33–58% Incidence of neonatal tetanus: 88–100%
Syphilis screening and treatment	IV	Prevalence-dependent
Preeclampsia and eclampsia: prevention (calcium supplementation)	IV	Prematurity: 34% (–1 to 57%) Low birthweight: 31% (–1 to 53%)

Contd...

Contd...

Intervention	Level	Effect
Intermittent presumptive treatment for malaria	IV	32% (−1 to 54%) PMR: 27% (1–47%) (first/second births)
Detection and treatment of asymptomatic bacteriuria	IV	Incidence of prematurity/low birthweight: 40% (20–55%)
Intrapartum		
Antibiotics for preterm premature rupture of membranes	IV	Incidence of infections: 32% (13–47%)
Corticosteroids for preterm labor	IV	40% (25–52%)
Detection and management of breech (cesarean section)	IV	Perinatal/neonatal death: 71% (14–90%)
Labor surveillance (including partograph) for early diagnosis of complications	IV	(early neonatal deaths): 40%
Clean delivery practices	IV	58–78% Incidence of neonatal tetanus: 55–99%
Postnatal		
Resuscitation of newborn baby	IV	6–42%
Breastfeeding	V	55–87%
Prevention and management of hypothermia	IV	18–42%
Kangaroo mother care (low birthweight infants in health facilities)	IV	Incidence of infections: 51% (7–75%)
Community-based pneumonia case management	V	27% (18–35%)

Interventions not included in evidence-based neonatal healthcare packages that are of benefit for infant, child, or maternal health

- Birth spacing
- Maternal zinc supplementation
- Maternal iron and folic acid supplementation
- Maternal iodine supplementation
- Neonatal vitamin A supplementation
- Insecticide-treated bed nets for malaria prevention
- Maternal antihelmintic treatment
- Prevention of maternal-to-child transmission of HIV
- Delayed umbilical cord clamping
- Prevention of ophthalmia neonatorum
- Hepatitis B vaccination and immunoprophylaxis

16. Millennium Development Goal (MDG)

Country or territory	Under-five mortality rate 1990	Under-five mortality rate 2006	Millennium Development Goal target 2015	Average annual rate of reduction (%) Observed 1990–2006	Average annual rate of reduction (%) Required 2007–2015	Progress towards the Millennium Development Goal target	Maternal mortality ratio (2005, adjusted)	Lifetime risk of maternal death (2005) 1in:	Level of maternal mortality
			Millennium Development Goal 4 (reduce by two-thirds, between 1990 and 2015, the mortality rate in children under age five)				Millennium Development Goal 5 (reduce by three-quarters, between 1990 and 2015, the maternal mortality ratio)[2]		
India	115	76	38	2.6	7.6	Insufficient	450	70	High

17.

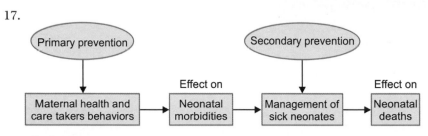

18. What works?

What can reduce neonatal deaths		
Intervention	*How it benefits*	*Potential impact (%)*
Tetanus toxoid injection during pregnancy	Prevents tetanus in newborn	33–58
Antibiotics for premature rupture of membrane	Reduces chances of infection in newborn	32
Corticosteroid treatment for preterm labor	Matures lungs of newborn	40
Partograph use	Management of delivery	40
Clean delivery	Reduces chances of infection in newborn	58–78
Resuscitation of newborn	Asphyxia management	6–42
Breastfeeding	Multiple benefits	55–87
Warmth to newborn	Hypothermia prevention	1.8–42
Community-based pneumonia management	Treatment of pneumonia	27

Source: Neonatal Survival Series 2: evidence-based, cost-effective interventions: how many newborn babies can we save? Lancet. 2005;365:977-88.

19. Birth day risk index (2013)

	Top 10 countries with the most first-day deaths	Number of first-day deaths	Share of global first-day deaths
1.	India	309,300	29%
2.	Nigeria	89,700	9%
3.	Pakistan	59,800	6%
4.	China	50,600	5%
5.	DR Congo	48,400	5%
6.	Ethiopia	28,800	3%
7.	Bangladesh	28,100	3%
8.	Indonesia	23,400	2%
9.	Afghanistan	18,000	2%
10.	Tanzania	17,000	2%
	Total	**673,200**	**64%**

20. The big five causes of stillbirths (http://www.thelancet.com/series/stillbirth, 2011):
    - Childbirth complications
    - Maternal infections in pregnancy
    - Maternal disorders, especially hypertension and diabetes
    - Fetal growth restriction
    - Congenital abnormalities

21. Four inexpensive under utilized lifesaving products:
    - Resuscitation equipment
    - Antenatal steroids
    - Chlorhexidine
    - Injectable antibiotics to treat sepsis/pneumonia.

SPOTS

Identify the symbol/spot

Sl. No	Spot	Comment
1.		Cochrane collaboration
2.		Biohazard

3.		National Rural Health Mission (NRHM)
4.		United Nations International Children Fund (UNICEF)
5.		World Health Organization (WHO)
6.		International Liaison Committee on Resuscitation (ILCOR)
7.		Transcutaneous bilirubinometer
8.		Mouth-to-mask resuscitator

9.		Oropharyngeal airway
10.		Oxygen reservoir
11.		Portable hand-held suction
12.		Nasopharyngeal airway
13.		Portable hand-held suction
14.		Portable hand-held suction device (Penguin model)
15.		Defibrillator

16.	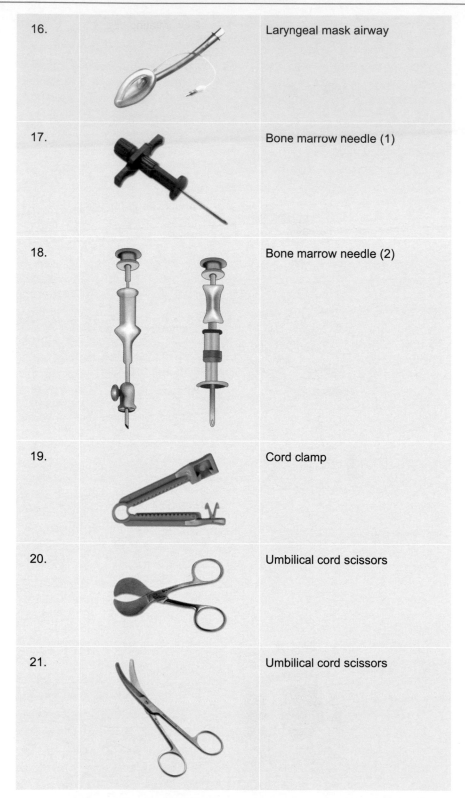	Laryngeal mask airway
17.		Bone marrow needle (1)
18.		Bone marrow needle (2)
19.		Cord clamp
20.		Umbilical cord scissors
21.		Umbilical cord scissors

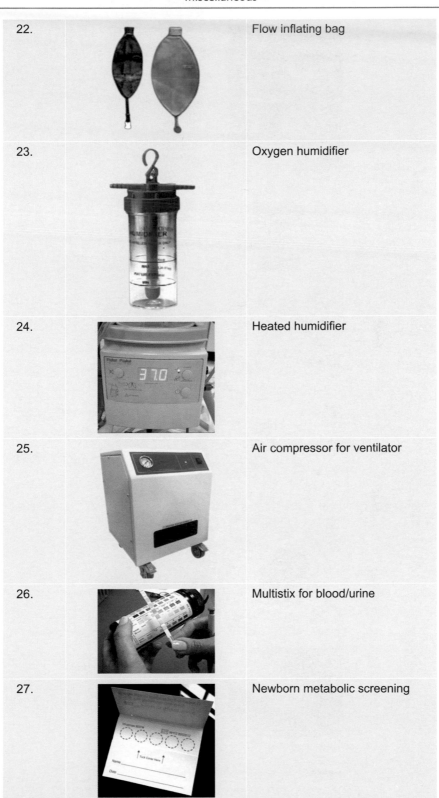

22.		Flow inflating bag
23.		Oxygen humidifier
24.		Heated humidifier
25.		Air compressor for ventilator
26.		Multistix for blood/urine
27.		Newborn metabolic screening

28.		Otoacoustic emissions (OAE) screening
29.		C-reactive protein (CRP) latex kit
30.		Band neutrophil
31.		Dohle bodies
32.		Toxic granules
33.		Capillary tube
34.		Intercostal drain

35.	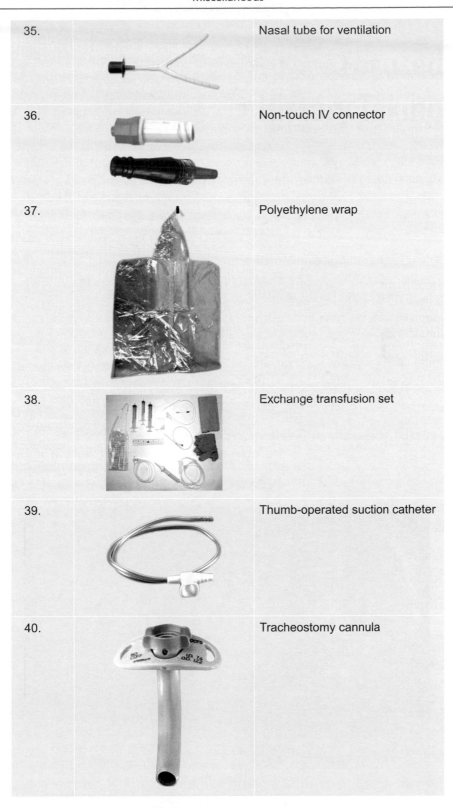	Nasal tube for ventilation
36.		Non-touch IV connector
37.		Polyethylene wrap
38.		Exchange transfusion set
39.		Thumb-operated suction catheter
40.		Tracheostomy cannula

41.		T piece connector
42.		Neonatal cooling therapy: Mira Cradle, phase changing material
43.		Transparent adhesive device
44.		Elastic adhesive bandage
45.		Nasal continuous positive airway pressure (CPAP) prong set (Hudson)
46.		Face mask
47.		Test lung (1)
48.		Test lung (2)

49.		Nasal prong (Argyle)
50.		Pneumothorax tray
51.		Disposable BP cuff
52.		Disposable pulse-oximeter probe
53.		Urine collection bag
54.		Disposable bacterial filter
55.		Microdrip set

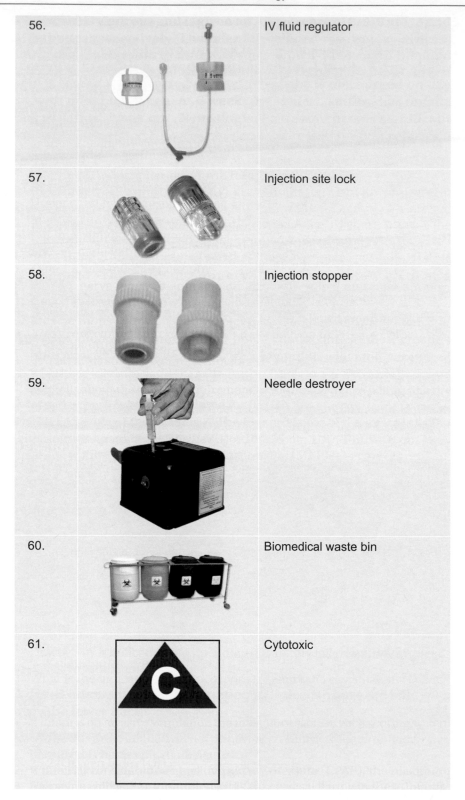

56.		IV fluid regulator
57.		Injection site lock
58.		Injection stopper
59.		Needle destroyer
60.		Biomedical waste bin
61.		Cytotoxic

62.	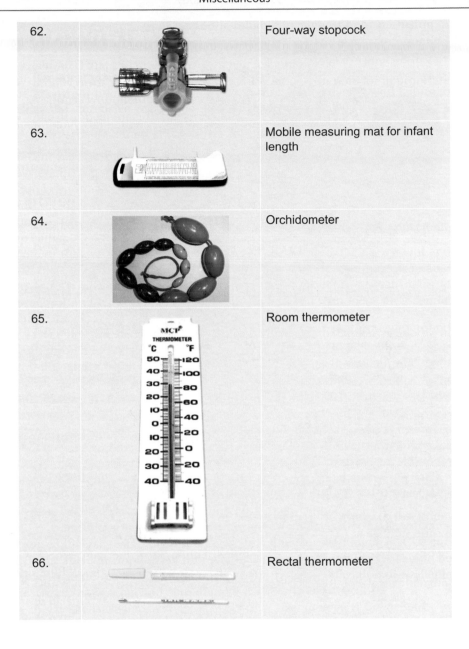	Four-way stopcock
63.		Mobile measuring mat for infant length
64.		Orchidometer
65.		Room thermometer
66.		Rectal thermometer

INDEX

Page numbers followed by *f* refer to figure.

A

Abdominal distension 166
Abdominal X-ray 242
Abnormal
    movements
        stabilize the neonate 42
        evaluate for 42
        identify the problem 43
        intervene 43
    patterns 33
    shoulder tone, clinical significance of
        22
    tone 8
Achondroplasia trisomy 21 30
Acidosis 86
Acrocyanosis 101
Active tone 21
Activity, general examination of
    newborn 8
Acute bilirubin encephalopathy 89
Acyl carnitine profile 48
Adduct the baby's hip 15
Adequacy of feeds 3
Air
    compressor for ventilator 273
    entry 29
Alae nasi 30, 45
Aldosterone deficiency 72
Alprostadil 142
Ambiguous genitalia 187
Amino acid metabolism 91
Amniotic fluid index 195
Amniotic fluid volume 36
Anastomotic leaks 160
Animal milk 45
Anogenital anomalies 10
Antenatal
    care 264*f*
    scan 247
    steroids 36, 173
Anterior
    fontanel 31
    superior iliac spine 15

Anteroposterior diameter 31
Anthropometry 8, 9
Antiglobulin 85
Antiretroviral 75
Antithyroid medication 113
Apgar score 26, 28
Apnea 9, 10, 28, 36-38, 40
Apneic 249
Appropriate for gestational age 41
Arterial blood gas 186
Arthrogryposis 14, 81
Assess for seizures 41
Assessing fontanel 31
Assessing hydration 43
    anterior fontanel 43
    breathing 44
    capillary refill 44
    eyes 43
    feeding 44
    mucous membrane 43
    pulse 44
    sensorium 43
    skin turgor 44
    urine flow 44
    weight 43
Asymmetric tonic neck reflex 25
Athetoid cerebral palsy 24
Audible sound 45
Autosomal dominant inheritance 215*f*
Autosomal recessive 60, 90, 91, 94, 100
Autosomal recessive inheritance 216*f*
Axonal neuropathy 60

B

Baby's
    abdomen 18
    blood group 53
    blood sample 53
    change in behavior 32
    chest 19
    eyes 11
    grip 22
    head 31
    heart rate 149

hip 15
palm 22
respiratory rate 190
Band neutrophil 274
Barlow test 15
Barlows-Otolarni 10
Barrel chest 38
Barter syndrome 3, 70
Basal ganglia region 181
Baseline tests 48
Beginning 1
Bell's stages of necrotizing enterocolitis
    104
Benign
    neonatal sleep myoclonus 43
    sleep myoclonus 43
Bevacizumab 115
Bifidobacteria 139
Bilateral cystic kidney disease 98
Bilateral fetal hydronephrosis 247
Bilateral hypointensive cystic 179
Bilateral intrauterine lesion 18
Bilateral pulmonary branch stenosis 59
Bilateral renal agenesis 98
Bile stones 7
Bilious vomiting 166
Bilirubin albumin molar ratio 86
Bilirubin staining 181
Biohazard 269
Biomedical waste bin 278
Biotinidase deficiency 91
Birth day risk index 269
Birth history 1
Bleeding tendency 39, 42
Blood collections 37
Blood pressure measurement 14
Bone marrow needle 272
Boot-shaped heart sign 65
Borderline personality disorder 253
Bosentan 65
Bounding pulses 174
Brachial plexus lesion 18
Brain malformation 18
Breastfeeding, assessment for 10
Breathing 9, 48
Bronchopulmonary dysplasia 169
Bronchoscopy 156
Bruises 17
Bubble CPAP settings, check for
    adequacy of 30
Bulging fontanel 31, 42

C

Calcaneovalgus foot 14
Capillary refill time 13
Capillary tube 274
Carbidopa 43
Cardinal points 10
Cardiogenic shock 40
Cardiotocogram 193
Cardiotocography 186
Cardiovascular system 29
Case studies
    adopted baby 106
    baby is pale with dysmorphism 59
    baby vaginal born, case 3 60
    cardiology 64
    day-6-infant on routine evaluation,
      electrolyte disturbances 68
    emergency and critical care 101
    gastroesophageal reflux 107
    inborn errors of metabolism 89
    infections in the newborn 73
    jaundice 82
    kangaroo care 61
    musculoskeletal 78
    necrotizing enterocolitis 104
    nephrology 97
    nutrition and growth 94
    retinopathy of prematurity screening
      113
    statistics 120
    thyroid disorders in the newborn 110
Center the baby's head 32
Central nervous system 30, 47
Cephalhematoma 17
Cerebellar nuclei 87
Cerebral palsy 18
Cervical cord lesion 18
Cherry red macular spot 90
Chest indrawing 44
Chest rise adequate 30
Chlorhexidine 14
Chorioamnionitis 36
Chorioretinitis 42
Choroid plexus cyst 176
Chronic
    constipation 244
    illness 36
Circulatory collapse, signs of 44
Clavicle 18
Clinical diagnosis of DDH, management
    of child 63

Clinical examination, focused 8-34
    blood pressure measurement 14
    breastfeeding, assessment for 10
    capillary refill time 13
    circumference measurement 11
    development dysplasia of hip 14
    head to toe physical examination 9
    heel to ear examination 19
    jaundice 16
    length 11
    popliteal examination 18
    scare sign 19
    weight 11
    well baby examination 8
Clonazepam 43
Cochrane collaboration 269
Cold stress 8, 101
Community-based pneumonia 267
Complete blood picture 87
Congenital adrenal hyperplasia 3, 47
Congenital cystic adenomatoid
    malformation 171
Congenital diaphragmatic hernia 187
Congenital fibular hemimelia 82
Congenital heart disease 8
Congenital hypertrophic pyloric stenosis
    45
Congenital hypothyroidism 31, 110
Congenital nephrotic syndrome 98
Congestive cardiac failure 101
Connatal cyst 175
Consanguinity 3, 41
Consciousness 8
Consent for
    new drug or trial 256
    therapeutic hypothermia 257
Continuous positive airway pressure 30
Contralateral hip 15
Cord clamp 272
Cortical blindness 180
Corticosteroids for preterm labor 267
Cough in a neonate
    assessment and plan 48
    counsel parents 49
    focused clinical examination 48
    focused history 48
    stabilize and assess 48
Counseling 253
Counseling steps 253
Cradle hold 10*f*
Craniosynostosis 31
Critical congenital heart disease 62
Cry 8

Crying 31
Cyanosis 8, 10, 29, 156
Cystic periventricular leukomalacia 175
Cytotoxic 278

D

Dandy-Walker syndrome 181
Danger signs 8, 10, 40
Death of baby
    after prolonged hospital stay 259
    elbw baby 258
    operated for diaphragmatic hernia
        260
Deep tendon reflexes 33
Defibrillator 271
Dehydration 44
    etiology 44
    identify cause for 44
Delayed capillary refill 44
Delivery care 264*f*
Denver developental screening test 26,
    197
Dermal sinus 248
Developmental dysplasia of hip 14
Diabetes insipidus 30, 68
Diarrhea 45
Diastematomyelia 81
Difficult labor 41
DiGeorge 59
Digoxin 65
Direct Coombs' test 37
Dislocated hip 15
Disposable
    bacterial filter 277
    BP cuff 277
    pulse-oximeter probe 277
Disseminated intravascular coagulation
    261
Distal heart sounds 39
Distal renal tubular acidosis 71
Dohle bodies 274
Dorsum of hands 22
Double bubble sign 164
Downe's score 28, 29
Drowsy 8
Drug withdrawal 43
Drugs 124
    adenosine 124
    adrenaline 125
    alpostin 142
    amphotericin 127
    anti-D 128

betamethasone 137
calcium gluconate 128
dexamethasone 136
dextrose 129
diazoxide 129
erythromycin 125
fluconazole 132
fosphenytoin 132
intravenous immunoglobulin 133
linezolid 133
low molecular weight heparin 134
lyophilized amphotericin 126
magnesium sulfate 125
milrinone 130
nitric oxide 135
normal saline 136
phenobarbitone 139
probiotics 139
propranolol 138
sildenafil 140
thiamine 128
vancomycin 141
Duchenne-Erb palsy 62
Ductus venosus 64
Duodenal stenosis 164
Dusky 8
Dysmorphism 17
Dysmotility 160
Dysplasia of hip 15

E

Ears 9
Ebstein's anomaly 66, 67
Echogenic medullary pyramids 69
Echymosis 37
Egg on string sign 65
Elastic adhesive bandage 276
Electrochemical sensors 144
Electroencephalography 42
Emergency assessment 35
Enterocolitis—sepsis 244
Erythroblastosis 16
Estimated stillbirth rate 262
Euvolemia 68
Evaluate tone patterns 32
Evidence-based interventions for
    mother and child
    antenatal 266
    intrapartum 267
    postnatal 267
    preconception 266
Excessive crying
    examination 45

history 45
    identify "danger signs" 45
Exchange transfusion set 275
Extended spectrum betalactamase 74
Extrauterine life 63
Extremely low birth weight 169
Eyes 9

F

Face mask 276
Facilitator instructions to 1
Facility-based newborn care 263
Falciform ligament 77
Fanconi's anemia 82
Fatty acid oxidation defects 47
Faulty feeding 44
Feeding history taking 2
Femoral pulses 48
Fetal
    distress 6, 41, 47
    growth restriction 262
    monitoring 3
Figure of 8 153
Flex hips 15
Flex lower limb 15
Flow inflating bag 273
Folic acid supplementation 266
Forearm recoil 21
Four-way stopcock 279
Functional residual capacity 27

G

Galactosemia 3, 7, 90, 91, 92
Galeazzi sign 15
Gallbladder removal 7
Gastroesophageal reflux 107
Gastroesophageal reflux disease 185
Gastrographin 71
Gastrointestinal tract 30
Gaucher's disease 92
Genetic disorder 81
Genitalia 9
Genitals 48
Gestation 8, 9, 32
Glucose insulin rate 207
Glucose-6-phosphate dehydrogenase 37
Glutaric aciduria 184
Glycogen storage disorders 47
Gonococcemia 78
Graf angle 63
Graves' disease 112, 113
Grunt 10
Grunting 28, 29

H

Hammersmith neonatal neurological 31
examination of 32
Head 9
control 32
in line with the body 10
to toe physical examination 9
Heated humidifier 273
Heel to ear examination procedure 19
Hematogenous spread 74
Hepatosplenomegaly 42
Hernial orifice 46
Hippocampus 87
Hips 10
Hirschsprung's disease 166, 244
Homocystinuria 90
Horizontal suspension 21
Humidification 30, 31
Hydranencephaly 18
Hydrocephalous 31, 175
Hydrops fetalis 85
Hyperekplexia 43
Hypertonia of neck extensors 22
Hypertrophic obstructive
cardiomyopathy 178
Hypertrophic pyloric stenosis 156
Hypochloremic 157
Hypoglycemia 5, 43, 90
assessment of hypoglycemic neonate
40
evaluation for sugar 5
feeding pattern 5
intrapartum asphyxia 6
intrapartum glucose infusion 5
maternal diabetes 5
maternal drugs 6
sepsis risk 6
Hypopigmented patches 42
Hypoplastic left heart syndrome 67
Hypotension 40
Hypothermia 8, 39, 43
Hypovolemic shock 40
Hypoxic
brain injury 43
ischemic encephalopathy 43, 251
ischemic injury 31

I

Icterus 42
Ileal atresia 166
Imaging
echocardiogram 176
interpretation of chest X-ray/
abdomen 153
differential diagnosis 154
indications for surgery in NEC
155
magnetic resonance imaging 179
neonatal cranial ultrasound 171
Immune globulin therapy 85
Imperforate anus 244
In vitro fertilization 257
Inadequate breast milk 4
Inborn errors of metabolism 254
India Newborn Action Plan (INAP) 2014
262
Infections in the newborn 73
Inferior vena cava 170
Injection site lock 278
Injection stopper 278
Institutional deliveries 266*f*
Instrument
bilirubinometer 143
FiO$_2$ monitor 144
fluxmeter 144
infusion pump 146
multichannel monitor 147
neonatal incubator 145
phototherapy unit 148
pulse oximeter 148
radiant warmer 149
self-inflating bag and mask 150
syringe pump 151
weighing machine 152
Intact interventricular septum 66
Intercostal drain 274
Intermittent positive pressure
ventilation 165
International Liaison Committee on
Resuscitation, symbol of 270
Interpretation
arterial blood gas 186
capnography 191
c-reactive protein 192
cardiotocography 193
Interpretation
Denver developemtal screening test-
II, reports of
Interpretation
genetics 210
hepatobiliary case studies 220
interpret the clinical picture 221
intrauterine growth chart 219
jaundice evaluation 224

286

using AAP jaundice management
chart for phototherapy 224
using hour specific bilirubin
prediction chart 225
micro erythrocyte sedimentation rate
227
neonatal electroencephalogram 200
neonatal surgery 241
neurology case studies 227
partograph 232
peripheral smear 234
pulmonary graphics 237
pulse oximeter predischarge 239
shake test 240
Intracranial hemorrhage 18
Intracranial pressure 31
Intrauterine infection
cocaine 41
heroin 41
maternal fever 41
maternal intake of alcohol 41
methadone 41
Ipsilateral decreased air entry 39
Ipsilateral ear 19
Irregular breathing 60
Isolated cleft palate 10, 39

J

Jaundice 16
assess of day 3 6
case studies
examination for newborn 16
extent of 16
neonatal 7
severity focused examination 36
severity focused investigations 37
staining the palms 16
Jaw myoclonus 43
Jitteriness 41-43

K

Kangaroo
mother care 267
position 61
Kernicterus 181
Klebsiella 73
Klebsiella sepsis 179
Klisic's test 15
Knees 15

L

Lactobacilli 139
Large caput 38

Large for gestational age 41
Laryngeal mask airway 272
Learner 1
Left hip joint 79
Left intraventricular hemorrhage 173
Lethargic 8
Lethargy 57
Levenes ventricular index 174
Levodopa 43
Levosimendan 65
Limb anamolies 82
Limbs 9
Listeria infection 75
Live births 262
Liver biopsy 221
Liver echotexture 87
Liver function tests 220
Low segment cesarean section 255
Lower limb posture 32
Lymphadenopathy 41

M

Maisels charts 86
Mann Whitney U test 123
Maternal
antihelmintic treatment 267
blood group 50
depression 3
fever 36
history 2
iron and folic acid supplementation
267
polyhydramnios 167
risk factors 2
zinc supplementation 267
Measurement of
head circumference 12, 13
length 12
equipment 11
procedure 11
weight 12
Mechanical ventilation 189
Meconium
aspiration syndrome 165, 177
liquor 6
stained amniotic fluid 250
staining 3, 38
Meningitis 31
Meningocele 14
Mental development 70
Metabolic acidosis 71, 89, 91, 92, 105,
128, 132, 155, 186, 190
Metatarsus adductus 14

Methylmalonic academia 90, 94
Microdrip set 277
Micturating cystourethrogram 97, 170
Midline defects 17
Millennium development goal 268
Milrinone 65
Mira cradle 276
Mitochondrial
   disorders 89
   inheritance 219
Mobile measuring mat for infant length
   279
Moro examination 17
Moro's reflex 17
Mortality with birth size 265
Mosaicism 211
Mother's
   abdomen 10
   age at the time of birth 264*f*
   breast 11*f*
Mouth 9
Mouth-to-mask resuscitator 270
Movements 33
Multifocal clonic movements 43
Multiple
   carboxylase deficiency 91
   organ dysfunction syndrome 252
Multistix for blood/urine 273
Murmur 38
Myelodysplasia 81
Myotonic dystrophy 60

N

Nasal continuous positive airway
   pressure 276
Nasal flaring 28
Nasal prong 277
Nasal tube for ventilation 275
Nasopharyngeal airway 271
Nasopharynx 78
National Rural Health Mission 270
Necrotizing enterocolitis 154
Needle destroyer 278
Neonatal
   and childhood illness 263
   cooling therapy 276
   deaths in India, causes of 263
   deaths, what can reduce 268
   mortality rate 262
   reflexes 17
   resuscitation, demonstrate 249
   chest compression 251
   management of meconium,
      stained amniotic fluid baby
      250
   positive pressure ventilation 249
   routine care 249
  vitamin A supplementation 267
Neonate's abdomen 10
Neurocutaneous markers 42
Neurogenic
   shock 40
   defects 18
Neuronal necrosis 181
Newborn
   general examination of 8
   intensive care unit 253
   metabolic screening 273
Nonoptimal 25
Non-touch IV connector 275

O

Observe tone and posture 32
Observed station 249
Obstructive shock 40
Occult congenital anomalies 10
Occult congenital anomaly 8
Oligohydraminos 15, 100
Ominous sign 40
Opisthotonus 22, 89
Optimal 32
Orchidometer 279
Organic academia 91
Orientation 33
   arousability and consolability 33
   visual orientation 33
Oropharyngeal airway 271
Oropharynx 78
Ortalani test 15
Oscillometry 14
Osteomyelitis 78
Osteopenia 168
Otoacoustic emissions screening 274
Overall evaluation of the learner 1
Oxygen
   humidifier 273
   reservoir 271

P

Palate 9
Pale mottled skin 44
Pallor 85
Palmar grasp reflex 22

Palpable lump 46
Paroxysmal tonic upgaze of childhood 43
Partograph 268
Passive tone 20
Patent ductus arteriosus 178
Pavlik harness 63, 79
Pelvis 15
Perform
    general observation 14
    lower limb examination 15
Perfusion 9
Perinatal
    asphyxia 175
    history
        natal 3
        postnatal 3
        prenatal 3
Peripheral smear 37
Peripherally inserted central catheter 170
Periventricular hemorrhagic infarction 173
Perpendicular 11
Petechiae 16, 39
Phenobarbital administration 251
    preparation 251
    steps of administration 252
Phenobarbitone 42, 251
Phenylephrine 116
Photophobia 118
Place heels 15
Plagiocephaly 14
Plantar grasp reflex 24, 25f
Plethora 8, 16
Pleural effusions 85
Pneumatosis intestinalis 166
Pneumonia 39
Pneumothorax 175, 277
Polycythemia 8
Polyethylene wrap 275
Polyhydramnios 3, 47
Polyuria 44, 45, 69
Poor weight gain evaluate for systemic causes of 29
Popliteal 32
Popliteal angle 32
    assess the tone of the hamstring muscles 18
    measuring 19f
Portable hand-held suction device 271
Positive pressure ventilation 249
Potter facies 38

Potter's syndrome 98
Prelacteals 4
Premature rupture of membranes 41
Preterm
    admission at birth 1
    babies 94
    infant 190
    labor 36
    premature rupture of membrane 186
Previous sibling unexpected death 255
    examination 48
    history 47
Primary pulmonary hypertension 177
Primigravida mother 50, 51, 83
Primitive reflexes 21
Prolonged labor 6
Prompt 1
Proparacaine 117
Pseudohypoaldosteronism 72
Pulmonary
    atresia 62, 66
    edema 168
    hemorrhage 168, 189
Pulse oximeter 9, 35
    predischarge 62
    screening 62
Pustules 39
Pyruvate dehydrogenase deficiency 89

R

Radial hemimelia 82
Rashtriya Bal Swasthya Karyakram 263
Rectal thermometer 279
Recurrent infections 3
Reflexes 33
Reporting of meta-analysis 121
Respiratory distress 4, 85
    case studies 53
    physical assessment 37
    scoring 27
    syndrome 168
Retinitis pigmentosa 90
Retinopathy of prematurity 253
Retractions 29
Retrocollis 22
Rh negative pregnancy 49
Rhabdomyolysis 72
Rigler sign 77
Robertsonian translocation 211
Rockerbottom foot 81

Room thermometer 279
Routine tracheal intubation 251

S

Sacral dimple 61
Salt wasting state 73
Salvia 242
Sandifer syndrome 43
Scaphoid abdomen 39, 161
Scarf sign
    assessment of shoulder tone 20
    normal parameters for shoulder tone
        evaluation 21
    procedure 20
    raise to sit and back to lying
        maneuver 21
Sclerema 39
Sensorium of baby 23
Sepsis
    calculate 122
    signs of 17
    symptoms of 16
Septic
    arthritis 78
    shock 40
Serum alkaline phosphatase 168
Serum ionic calcium 42
Severe gastroesophageal reflux 71
Severe perinatal asphyxia 18
Shallow breathing 44
Shock
    asphyxia, risk of 5
    assessment for 39
    bleeding per vaginal 5
    feeding 5
    losses 5
    sepsis risk 5
Shoulder tone in newborn 20
Sick babies 16
Sick newborn
    case studies 56-57
    identifying 35
Sildenafil 65
Silverman Andersen score 27, 28
Slanting palpebral fissures 210
Sleep 3
Small for gestational age 41
Smooth brain 184
Snowman 153
Soft palate dysfunction 59
Spastic
    cerebral palsy 23
    hemiplegia 24

quadriparesis 180
    type 18
Specific test 15
Spina bifida 14
Spinal
    cord injury 23
    defects 10
    dysraphism 14
    muscular atrophy 60
Splenectomy 7
Splenomegaly 37
Spontaneous 2
    abnormal movements 33
    perforation 154
Spots, identify symbols/spot 269-279
Stabilization 35, 42
Staphylococcus aureus 74
Staphylococcus epidermidis 76
Startle 33
Stepping and placing 33
Stool pattern 3
Subependymal cyst 175
Subgaleal bleeds 42
Suboptimal 32
Substantia nigra 87
Sucking reflex 33
Sudden death 47
    neonatal death in unit 254
    newborn in the unit 255
Sunken fontanel 31
Supravalvular aortic stenosis 59
Swollen scrotum 46
Symptomatic anemia 85
Syphilis 3, 266
Syphilitic arthritis 78

T

Tachycardia 85, 174, 175
Tachypnea 44, 53, 85
Tay–Sachs disease 90
Tecotherm 258
Test abduction 15
Test lung 276
Testing 32
Tetanus toxoid
    immunization 266
    injection 268
Tetralogy of Fallot 62, 67
The State of World's Children, WHO,
    2012 266
Thrombocytopenia 36, 82, 155
Thumb-operated suction catheter 275
Thyroid scintiscanning 185

Thyroxine binding globulin 111
Tone at elbow 32
Torticollis 14
Total anomalous pulmonary venous
    return 177
Total parenteral nutrition 3
Total serum bilirubin 16
Toxic granules 274
Toxoplasmosis 3, 74
T piece connector 276
Tracheoesophageal fistula 48, 167
Tracheostomy cannula 275
Transcutaneous bilirubinometer 270
Transient tachypnea 159
Transillumination test 166
Transparent adhesive device 276
Tremors 33
Tricuspid
    atresia 62
    valve regurgitation jet 177
Trisomy syndromes 17
Trochanter 15
Tropicamide 114, 116
Truncus arteriosus 62
Trunk in ventral suspension 32
Twins 3, 6, 39
Tyrosinemia type 1 91
Tzanck test 78

U

Ulnar aspect 22
Ultrasound abdomen 220
Umbilical
    arterial catheter 163
    cord scissors 272
Unconsolable cry 45
Underlying artery 14
Unexplained
    birth asphyxia 252
    neonatal deaths 6
United Nations International Children
    Fund 270
Unstable vital parameters 16
Unwell 35
Upper limb 32
Urine collection bag 277
Urine output 3

V

Vaccination 36
Vaginal delivery 4, 82, 83
Varicella infection 76
Velocardiofacial syndrome 59
Ventilator settings, check for adequacy
    of 30
Ventriculomegaly 174
Vertical suspension 21
Vesicoureteral reflux 99
Vigevano maneuver 43
Vitals 8
Vitamin K 36
Vitamins for neonatal cholestasis 222
Volume overload states 68
Vomiting 30, 31, 45
    examination 47
    exclude emergency first 46
    history 47
VQ scan 156

W

Waiter' tip 62
Warmth to newborn 268
Weak cry 40
Weak rapid pulse 44
Weighing machine 152
Weight
    gain pattern 45
    length and occipitofrontal
        circumference 11
    loss 16, 44
Well baby examination 8
Wet 46
Whole body 10
Williams syndrome 59
Wire-vectis 116
Work of breathing 40
World Health Organization 270
Worsening sensorium 40

X

Xiphisternum 61
Xiphoid retractions 28
X-linked 93
    dominant inheritance 218
    recessive 217
X-ray limbs 75*f*

Z

Zellweger syndrome 92, 184